Praise for
Aspertools . . .

"I strongly recommend Dr. Reitman's book *Aspertools* to people who are interested in understanding that each child is entitled to learn and develop in a way that enables that child to succeed. . . ."

—**Abraham Fischler**
President Emeritus, Nova Southeastern University

"I believe that *Aspertools* by Dr. Hackie Reitman is at the vanguard of changing peoples' perceptions about what's going on with our brains."

—**Brian Udell, M.D.**
Medical Director, The Child Development Center of America

"*Aspertools* will help in so many ways. Without realizing it, Dr. Hackie Reitman has written a great book about *all* relationships and parenting."

—**Dr. Lori J. Butts, J.D., Ph.D.**
President, Florida Psychological Association, 2015,
Director of the Clinical and Forensic Institute

"*Aspertools* brings hope and optimism to Aspies and their families! After so many books filled with diagnostic tools and statistical data, *finally*, here is a book about Asperger's syndrome that actually offers something helpful: how to cope with the various symptoms and overcome the challenges. The insight and practical advice from the multiple points of view—the Aspie, the parent, and the educator—provide a comprehensive yet easily readable work. Thank you, Dr. Reitman, for reaffirming that Aspies *can* and *do* lead productive, fulfilling lives!"

—**Delfina B.**
Aspie mom

"What an awesome story of impact and vision! On behalf of the 'KID' in all of us, thanks."

—**Mark D. Dhooge**
President/CEO, Kids In Distress, Inc.

"As a professor of philosophy, I have taken some instruction from *Aspertools*. Dr. Reitman has given me a more profound grasp of the fact that one size does not fit all when it comes to learning, and that what one student can handle with aplomb might cause another to grind his teeth with anxiety."

—**Gordon Marino**
Professor of Philosophy at St. Olaf College,
editor of *The Quotable Kierkegaard,* and
writer, *The New York Times* and *The Wall St. Journal*

"When I read *Aspertools*, I thought, 'My gosh, Dr. Reitman is writing about my two teenagers!' This book has opened my eyes."

—**Dawn D.**
mother, medical technician

"*Aspertools* is a big help. I think too many people don't know enough about Asperger's, the autism spectrum, and different brains in general. . . . I think Dr. Hackie Reitman himself wishes he would've known these tools when his daughter was growing up."

—**Dr. Susan J. Mendelsohn**
clinical psychologist and life coach

ASPERTOOLS

The Practical Guide for Understanding and Embracing Asperger's, Autism Spectrum Disorders, and Neurodiversity

Harold S. Reitman, M.D.
with Pati Fizzano and Rebecca Reitman

Health Communications, Inc.
Deerfield Beach, Florida

www.hcibooks.com

Library of Congress Cataloging-in-Publication Data
is available through the Library of Congress

© 2014 Harold S. Reitman, M.D.

ISBN-13: 978-07573-1853-5 (Paperback)
ISBN-10: 07573-1853-3 (Paperback)
ISBN-13: 978-07573-1854-2 (ePub)
ISBN-10: 07573-1854-1 (ePub)

Publisher: Health Communications, Inc.
      3201 S.W. 15th Street
      Deerfield Beach, FL 33442–8190

Cover design by Larissa Hise Henoch
Interior design and formatting by Lawna Patterson Oldfield

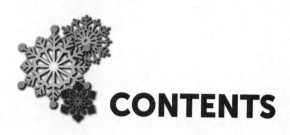

CONTENTS

Foreword vii

Acknowledgments xi

Preface: "Everyone's Brain Is Different" xix

Introduction: Who Am I Calling an Aspie? 1

1 Anxiety 7

2 Hypersenses: Senses on Steroids 15

3 Observation: "Elementary, My Dear Watson" ... 25

4 The Meltdown 31

5 The Safe Place 37

6 Rudeness, Truth Telling, and Manners 43

7 Transitions 51

8 Routines 57

9 Structure and Positive Activities 65

10 Obsessions and Hyper-Interests 71

11 Social Awkwardness 81

12 Limit Choices to Avoid "No!" 91

13 Instilling Street Smarts 97

14 Taking Things Literally: "Why Did They Say
I'm Not Playing with a Full Deck?" 105

15 Specifics: Say What You Mean,
Mean What You Say 113

16 Preventing Overwhelm: Breaking Down
Big Jobs into Smaller Tasks 119

17 Setting Goals 125

18 Rules, Rewards, and Consequences 131

19 Checklists: The Indispensable Tool 141

20 Time Management: Tools for Getting
Your Aspie to Be on Time 149

21 Overlapping Conditions 155

22 It's Not About You 161

23 Love Unconditionally 165

Afterword: Neurodiversity 169

Appendix A: A List of Aspertools 175

Appendix B: Advocacy 177

Appendix C: Resources 183

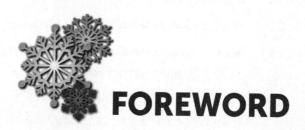

FOREWORD

Dr. Harold "Hackie" Reitman's *Aspertools* is a book that throws the book at stereotypes. However, before we get to the specifics, permit me to note that the author himself is someone who defies stereotypes. After all, Dr. Reitman is a former professional boxer who boasted a heavyweight right hand. He was also a renowned orthopedic surgeon, who used the same hands that produced hurt to remove it by repairing torn ligaments and bones. Again, he is not your stereotypical doctor or boxer, or, for that matter, author.

I first encountered Dr. Reitman in the corridors of boxing. I was writing a story about the legendary boxing trainer Angelo Dundee. Over time, I was blessed to develop a friendship with Angelo, and in our almost daily phone conversations he kept pestering me, "You have to meet my friend Hackie Reitman. You two would be great pals."

One does not become a Hall of Fame boxing trainer without being something of a master psychologist. Angelo was right; Hackie and I hit it off right away, in part because he is such a warm, compassionate, and open individual, which, by the way, are qualities that resonate throughout the pages you're about to turn.

In our first conversations, one of the issues that Hackie shared was his ongoing education about Asperger's. This was an education that he received slowly and often painfully as he came to understand that his daughter Rebecca was an "Aspie."

The good doctor struggled mightily to understand the landscape of Rebecca's mind and feelings. At one point, after Rebecca graduated from college, her father tried to push her along the career path of becoming a teacher. Resisting, Rebecca instructed him, "Everyone's brain is different. Brains are like snowflakes—no two are alike."

While it might seem like a contradiction, since this is a book of practical advice for people dealing with a distinct set of challenging thought and behavior patterns, Rebecca's observation that "No two brains are exactly alike" is perhaps the fulcrum of this book. The philosophical point (and there are many between these covers) is that with all the lush diversity of humankind, we have to be alive to the fact that some people experience the same thing in radically different ways.

For instance, in the first chapter "Anxiety," Hackie confides that there were times when he reacted angrily to Rebecca's reluctance to enter into seemingly social situations that he saw as only positive. He thought she was simply being stubborn. But then he came to understand that some people do not have a ready store of knowledge as to how to read and react to others. More likely than not, many of these same folks are also hypersensitive to ordinary stimuli such as light and noise.

After learning his lesson, a now enlightened Hackie realized that "a major source of anxiety for an Aspie is being placed in a social gathering or a new situation."

In the book, he prods us to imagine, "If you had to keep solving the same problems you solved the day before, if your every interaction with another human being seemed like rocket science, wouldn't you be anxious? And if you were always aware that your anxiety could escalate to a full meltdown, wouldn't that make you even more anxious?"

As a professor of philosophy, I have taken some instruction from *Aspertools*. Hackie has brought me to a more profound grasp of the facts that one size does not fit all when it comes to learning, and that what one student can handle with aplomb might cause another to grind his teeth with anxiety.

Moreover, the chapter on hyper-interests (more commonly known as "obsessions"), has helped me to be more patient with my students who come to a liberal arts college such as the one that I teach at, and nevertheless get locked into what seems like a rigid and limited set of subjects.

It is easy to preach about the importance of appreciating different ways of thinking, but this book practices what it preaches. At many junctures, we have the author's experience of a situation reflected on by a trained teacher of Aspies and then balanced by Rebecca's experience of the same. There are number of points at which Hackie presents us with a specific situation, followed by the mind- and heart-expanding exercise, "Imagine you are an Aspie."

Hackie Reitman is a perennial problem solver. There is little theory between these covers. This is preeminently practical Baedeker, brimming with vivid examples, sage counsel, and boundless good will.

—**Gordon Marino, Ph.D.**
Professor of Philosophy
Director, Hong Kierkegaard Library, St. Olaf College

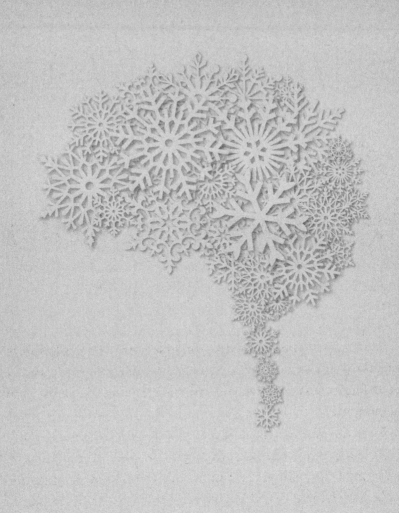

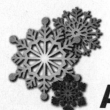

ACKNOWLEDGMENTS

In writing this book I am thankful to so many, and feel fortunate that this is the case. To those accidentally not mentioned I ask for your forgiveness and give you my thanks; please know that you are important.

First, thank you to my inspirational hero, my daughter Rebecca Reitman, to whom I dedicate this book. I love and admire her with all of my heart, all the time, no matter what. Rebecca walks the walk. I wish I had Rebecca's courage, brilliance, heart, and brain. I am so proud of her. She contributed greatly to this book with her unique insights from all sides of the learning table: as a gifted tutor-teacher for so many; as a role model for others; as a college graduate who understands her discrete mathematics degree from Georgia Tech; and as a daughter who admonishes me: "Dad, sometimes good intentions are not enough."

I am so grateful for Pati Fizzano's voice of experience, hope, and the kindness that she offers—with reason and results—to her students and their families. What a difference she has made as Rebecca's mentor, colleague, fellow teacher and tutor, and "family." In short, Pati "gets it." As she always says, "They can do it." Pati has helped so many students as a strategist and teacher, and contributed greatly to this book.

I thank and stand in the shadow of my parents, Ev and Phil, whose hard work and example enabled all four Reitman kids to make it in this world. My mother, Evelyn Goldberg Reitman, taught the eight-year-old version of me an important lesson one day as she was pumping gas at the family filling station in Jersey City: "You have a moral obligation to work up to your full potential with the gifts that G-d has given you, to help yourself, your family, your friends, and those less fortunate. And to have a good time doing it."

I thank my friend and mentor Tim Van Patten for his encouragement and teaching. Somehow he found the time to help me even as he was directing, writing for, and producing *The Sopranos*, *Boardwalk Empire*, and the like—while also tending to his wonderful family. I will always appreciate it. My first movie, *The Square Root of 2*, and this book became real in no small part because I accepted Tim's positive statement: "Hackie, no matter what anybody ever tells you, remember this: If you have a good story, with good characters, and good execution, it will make it. Don't let anybody discourage you."

I envy and have benefited from the loyalty and brilliance of David Linsley, who leads our wonderful young team here at PCE Media. Together, they surround this extremely lucky old man with their youthful insights and contributions: "Doc, this project is solid—all day long."

I am thankful for and remain stunned by the extraordinarily talented and hardworking actress Darby Stanchfield, who had the lead role in my movie production *The Square Root of 2*. Her method acting through direct study of Rebecca resulted in a nuanced portrayal of an honest young woman with challenges, including undiagnosed Asperger's syndrome. This fact was unknown—even to me—at the time of production, and it was this revelation later on that led me to write this book.

I am indebted to my cousin and first editor, Peter Bochner, for his loyalty and insistence on excellence and exactitude. His willingness to share his editing thought processes has definitely made me a better writer: "Hackie, you have that story wrong. Your mother, Ev, poured linguini with clam sauce on my head, *not* spaghetti with meatballs—which I would have eaten."

I needed and greatly appreciate the opportunity and excellent professional support given to me by the professional staff at Health Communications, Inc. (HCI), including Peter Vegso, Christian Blonshine, senior editor Christine Belleris (whose insightful and provocative manuscript queries made me dig deep!), and communications director Kim Weiss. What a great team! The HCI goal is to help people. Thanks for giving me a shot! I hope it's the first of many.

I appreciate and trust my irreplaceable lifetime friendship with Rebecca's "uncles," the Jersey City boys, Paul Kaliades, Jan Brody, Ken D'Elia, and Ken Kiken, who remind me: "Hack, you're still a moron."

I am thankful to and heed the wisdom of my longtime friend, CPA, and mentor Bernie Karcinell, who always makes me ask and answer the question: "What am I trying to accomplish?"

I thank and follow my boxing trainer-manager and friend Tommy Torino's metaphor for life. As he laced up my gloves before my first ten-round, pro heavyweight fight at the tender age of forty-one, he imparted these words of wisdom: "Just move forward throwing punches until the other guy falls down. Don't make it more complicated than that. That's all you can do."

I am lucky to have my friend and attorney since 1978, Steve Moody, looking over my shoulder, and keeping me out of trouble by often warning me, "Hack, you don't want to do that."

I thank Boston University's six-year medical program for taking a chance on a guy who had been expelled twice, (once in first grade, once in tenth grade) but knew he absolutely needed to become an MD. Also, I thank Dr. Robert E. Leach, Dr. Rich Paul, Dr. Thomas Einhorn, the Boston University Orthopaedic Residency Training Program, and the Boston University School of Medicine for allowing me to deliver my anatomy lecture to every first-year medical school class for thirty-six years.

I recognize each day the extrapolation of the teaching of orthopaedic surgery by trauma chief Dr. David Segal at Boston City Hospital, who taught me so well: "Take care of every emergency trauma patient from A to Z when they first come in, no matter what it takes. If you do everything with honesty and excellence, then every time you see them after that, it's just social visits."

I learned much from screenwriter Steve Greenberg, who lives the cinema: "It's just Screenwriting 101."

I admire eighty-seven-years-young Abe Fischler, President Emeritus of Nova Southeastern University, and his educational vision. I thank him for inspiring me: "I have to keep working, Hackie. The educational system is too important."

I try to emulate the faith and humor of my friend, the world's greatest strength and conditioning coach, Ian Pyka: "Which guy? The first guy or the second guy?"

I try to bring the good cheer and good wishes that my Uncle Moe brought to every human being he encountered: "Look, that's what happens. Don't worry about it anymore."

I attempt to be as upbeat and positive as Gretchen, who does it all for so many, every day, who reminds me: "You have so much to be thankful for. Everybody is healthy. You better get with the program and get happy."

I try to help others the way I see my friend Joey Esposito do so naturally: "Come to the front door, I have a surprise for you."

I am thankful for the existential writing coaching of my friend, philosophy professor Gordon Marino, who flat out told me: "Shut up and write the book already."

I recognize the constant, consistent, motherly love that Marilee has for Rebecca: I'm proud of you, Rebecca."

I still hear Beau Jack at the 5th Street Gym imploring me, commanding me to be my best: "Don't take a step backwards—ever."

I miss my friend, the late, great Bruce Rossmeyer, who did so much for so many while making it look easy. He'd see me struggling, pat me on the shoulder, then would smile and say: "Hackie, if it was easy, anybody could do it."

I thank Jane P. Singer and Bob Heyden. The chapter on hyperinterests, which focuses on my late friend, Charlie Singer, was improved significantly by Charlie's sister Jane, and Bob Heyden, Charlie's co-worker at Meadowlands Racetrack in New Jersey. They generously gave of their time for interviews in order to share memories of a brother and a friend. Charlie told me long, long ago: "No way was Mycroft smarter than Sherlock Holmes."

I thank Steve Forman, author of *Boca Knights*, for his friendship and for introducing me to his literary agent, Bob Diforio.

I am grateful for the guidance of my literary agent Bob Diforio: "I'll tell you the same thing I told Ken Follett when he asked me the same question. 'An author should write what he is passionate about and what he wants to write about, and not try to figure out what people want to read or what will be commercially viable.' "

I am proud of the children of the Hackie Reitman Club of The Boys and Girls Clubs of Broward County (in the toughest zip code in the country, 33311), such as Demetrius Brown, who prove the odds wrong every day: "Doc, I graduated today with two degrees from FSU."

I am grateful that I heard Angelo Dundee state his philosophy to me more than once: "It don't cost nothin' to be nice."

While still in medical school I confessed to one of the greatest heavyweight champions of all time, Joe Louis, at Caesars Palace that I got scared before every one of my Golden Gloves fights. I was stunned when he comforted me by saying: "Doc, we all take fear into the ring with us. It's what you do with it that makes you a champion."

I was relieved when Lem Banker told me the principle: "As long as you didn't ask him to take the punches for you, you can tell him where to go."

Thanks to Michelle Rubin (Autism after 21) and Jake Spooner, whose fateful meeting led me to HCI publisher Peter Vegso.

Thank you to all who shared their knowledge with me and motivated me, including Jaclyn Merens, Ana Brushingham, Kathleen Cohn, W. Bill Cohn, William Petri, Sarah Petri, Surah Corwin, Giovanna Epae, Reece Erlichman, and Wendy Van Patten.

I am thankful to all the students and interns—whether at Boston University, OAUSA, PCE Media, or anywhere else—for helping and inspiring me, and for allowing me to be of some help.

I apologize to all those great people to whom I owe so much, but whom my poor brain has forgotten to mention here. Please forgive me, but please accept my thanks: "I took too many shots to the head!"

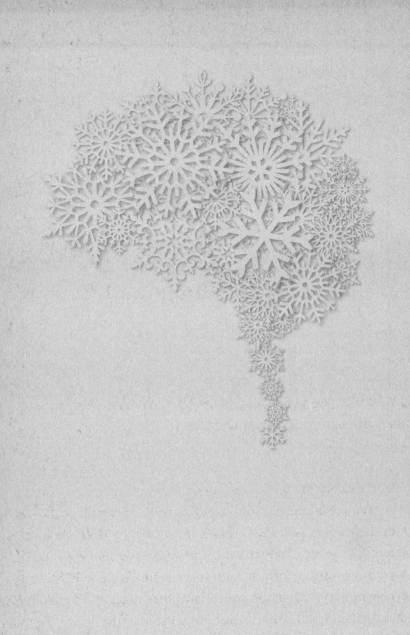

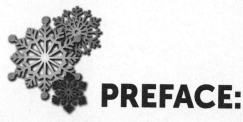

PREFACE:
"Everyone's Brain Is Different"

I never came upon any of my discoveries through
the process of rational thinking.

—*Albert Einstein*

Abe Fischler is an educational visionary and a friend of mine.
Abe was president of Nova Southeastern University in Davie,
Florida (west of Fort Lauderdale), from 1970 to 1992. Under his
leadership, Nova developed the first doctoral distance education
program—long before the Internet. Technology allowed it to
evolve into today's online educational programs. Today, Nova is
the eighth largest private university in the country.

Abe and I got to be friends when my daughter, Rebecca, was
attending the elementary school affiliated with Nova. I once asked
him what he thought the biggest problem was with our country's
educational system. He thought for a moment and said, "It's that

we take all of our students and put them in the same box simply because they have birthdays the same year."

That made me think of all I'd learned in every field of endeavor I had ever tried, including medicine, professional boxing, teaching, mentoring, writing, and movie and media production. Abe's observation applied to the individuals in all of them. For me, it was a "lightbulb moment." *One size does not fit all.* It *never* has. When it comes to teaching, learning, and training, it's an inconvenient fact for our educational system, the workplace, and even society as a whole.

Fast-forward a few decades. My daughter, Rebecca, received her degree in discrete mathematics[1] from the prestigious Georgia Institute of Technology, aka Georgia Tech, in 2009. She was one of the few women that year to earn her degree in this subject. This would have been quite an accomplishment under any circumstance but especially for her. Rebecca has twenty-three brain tumors, underwent two major brain surgeries at the Mayo Clinic when she was only a toddler, and had learning disabilities. This degree would have made her very valuable in the technology-driven job marketplace. However, shortly after receiving her diploma, she announced that she was going to stay in Atlanta and tutor math, one-on-one, to students with Asperger's syndrome, high-functioning autism, and other learning disabilities. From her years in middle school when she helped tutor other students (yes, she tutored other kids), she knew she wanted to work with learning-challenged children. She would assist these "different brain" kids from time to time, and not only did her students benefit greatly but she loved doing it. They loved her, too—they flocked to her for help.

I pressed her on her decision. "Rebecca, why not become a full-fledged teacher rather than a tutor? That way you'd be helping a whole classroom of students, and you'd have an actual career."

She shook her head, smiled, and sighed. "Dad, you just don't get it. Everyone's brain is different. Brains are like snowflakes—no two are alike. The kids I want to work with can't get the help they need in a classroom. They require one-on-one attention. And tutoring *is* going to be my career."

Rebecca was so right that day. Everyone's brain is different. She was also right about me— at least back then—not "getting it." Sadly, it would take me many more years to get it.

Helping others get it when it comes to those with Asperger's syndrome and similar "so-called" learning disabilities (*so-called* because today I think of them as simply different brains) is why I wrote this book. It wasn't until my daughter was well into her adulthood that I discovered Rebecca had Asperger's syndrome herself! It's also why I have delayed the release of *The Square Root of 2*, a movie inspired by the true story of a young woman with a seizure disorder and learning challenges going off to college, where she encounters—and fights—the school's unjust, one-size-fits-all system. It was only after I made the movie that I realized Rebecca had Asperger's! This realization inspired me to write this book.

I've gained a great deal of knowledge and insight about Asperger's syndrome over the past several years; if only I'd had it when my daughter was growing up. For most of her childhood, early adulthood, and all the way through her college years, I was just another well-intentioned parent who was clueless about Asperger's. Now that I finally have some insights about dealing with this developmental difference, I want to share them.

I am a medical doctor and spent my career as an orthopedic surgeon, but that has nothing to do with why I wrote this book. After all, what do doctors who deal with the musculoskeletal system know about this stuff? I'm writing this book not as a professional authority on Asperger's but as the parent of a child (who's now an adult) with Asperger's. I'm writing for other parents of children (or adults) who have Asperger's, autism, or any of the other neurological, psychological, or learning disability labels applied to individuals whose *brains are different*. I'm writing for teachers, professionals,[2] businesses, and the "Aspies" themselves. I guess when you get right down to it, I'm writing *Aspertools* for a pretty broad audience: all of society.

So who am I calling an Aspie? Anyone whose brain is a bit *different*, anyone who can benefit from the lessons I've learned from my ongoing education about Asperger's. Don't worry if the individual you care about does not truly have Asperger's syndrome or if some chapters in this book don't apply to that person. Just take the material that's of help. As a psychologist friend said, "Hackie, you may not realize it, but your book isn't just about Asperger's; it's a book on parenting and relationships in general." If the shoe fits, wear it. No need to get caught up in labels.

The truth is that we're talking about the neurological, electrical wiring system that determines our behavior. The brain inside our skulls—our living "personal" computer—has its own "hardware." And society seems to be trying to use the exact same "software" for every different brand of computer. If I were to try to run PC software on my Mac, I wouldn't get very far. Society has to see that the brains of its members can be quite different. In fact, they're getting more so as our central neurological structure undergoes a metamorphosis because of the demands that technology and our increasingly multitasking culture is placing upon us.

I think labels are a lousy way to describe a unique human being, whether we're talking about Asperger's, high-functioning autism, ADHD, ADD, ASD, or OCD, as well as giftedness, auditory or visual processing disorders, dyslexia, dyscalculia, executive functioning, depression, epilepsy, sensory integrative disorder, or Tourette's. One size does *not* fit all. Everybody's brain is different. Different methods can work for different brains. Abe Fischler's summation of the educational system's problem means that a group of kids the same age in the same classroom studying the same subject doesn't mean they need to learn the same way, at the same pace, with the same method. With the use of online learning technology and modern teaching techniques, we can all proceed at our own pace.

My daughter, Rebecca, is my hero. She's now in her thirties and, as she planned when she first graduated from Georgia Tech, is tutoring and mentoring a wide range of students whose brains are a bit different. She somehow managed to accomplish all this despite the cluelessness and missteps of her well-intentioned parents. Your Aspie (by that, I mean your individual who, among other traits, also happens to have a brain that works differently), no matter the age, deserves the same shot at maximizing his or her potential for independence and for living as any other person. And, dear reader, it's your job to spread that message to our greater society.

The educational system and the workplace, even society at large, need to embrace the fact that every brain is different and make that work to everyone's advantage. Leading-edge media and technology businesses are way ahead of America's old-fashioned, one-size-fits-all educational system and traditional brick-and-mortar companies when it comes to this. Apple, Google, and other companies are leading the way in recruiting and harnessing the brainpower of employees whose brains are different. So let's get real: neurodiversity is here to stay and, in fact, is a growing trend.

I didn't really begin to "get" what Rebecca had said about no two brains being alike until she began her post-graduate internship at an independent school in Atlanta for students with academic and social differences.

During a visit with Rebecca, I told the headmistress I was interested in making a documentary about the school. I asked if I could observe Rebecca's tutoring sessions and interview some of the students and parents. My real goal, however, was to learn more about learning challenges, particularly those related to Asperger's.

Rebecca didn't much care for her father hanging around, but she agreed to tolerate it as long as I didn't distract the students . . . particularly hers. That meant I couldn't do much filming or tape recording. But I did do a lot of observing of the academic environment. That's when I finally began to grasp what Rebecca meant when she said that these kids whose brains worked differently needed one-on-one attention.

For example, Billy was doing well in all his high school courses except math. Rebecca worked long hours with Billy, meeting with him individually and in a group, with his parents, and with his math teacher. Finally, Rebecca realized that Billy was a visual learner who needed to see things move physically to understand mathematical concepts. She and the teacher concluded that Billy was a kinesthetic learner; that is, when they taught him by moving objects around on a desk, he came up with the answer about half of the time. After further studying the situation, Rebecca discovered that if she moved the objects only from right to left, Billy got the answer right 100 percent of the time. Who else could have figured that out? Certainly not some so-called neurotypical[3] teacher in a big group classroom using one-size-fits-all teaching methods.

Today Rebecca is working with children who struggle with math at a middle school in Palm Beach County in South Florida. The school has an enrollment of 1,200 students, 30 of whom have Asperger's syndrome. Some of her students have so-called learning difficulties (but actually they're merely different). She continues to come up with creative tutoring solutions to help them understand the material. She works alongside Pati Fizzano, who teaches, and truly understands, students with Asperger's. Pati is certified as an Exceptional Student Education (ESE) and autism spectrum disorder (ASD) teacher who has been involved in the Asperger's community for many years. She has been coaching Rebecca and has made Rebecca her protégé.

One middle school student was a distraction to everyone. Bobby wouldn't sit still in class and wanted nothing to do with math. Rebecca was asked to evaluate the situation. After a series of meetings with Bobby, his parents, and his teacher, Rebecca brought him alone into a study room for his first tutoring session. Bobby was distraught and could not stop pacing back and forth. Rebecca asked him to have a seat. He grudgingly took a chair but kept looking side to side, wringing his hands, and tugging at his hair. Even after Rebecca announced the session was starting, he couldn't focus on any of the math concepts she was trying to convey. Realizing the situation wasn't working, she asked Bobby, "Do you want to sit, or would you rather pace?"

Bobby looked at Rebecca in disbelief. "You mean I can pace while I do these problems and go through the lessons?"

Rebecca smiled. "Sure. If it will help you learn."

It did.

Another problem student was Devin, a brilliant teen who hated doing math homework. No teacher could get him to stop listening to his iPod or watching videos on his phone. But Rebecca offered Devin a deal: he could play his music and watch his videos if he simultaneously did his math homework. Devin agreed and soon was doing his homework in an unorthodox multitasking environment that no other teacher or tutor would have considered—let alone allowed.

Why did Rebecca allow Bobby to pace back and forth and Devin to listen to music while she was tutoring them? Because she asked a simple question: What am I trying to accomplish?[4] And in each of these cases, it was not putting a student in a traditional tutoring environment but getting them to learn math concepts successfully, consistently, and effectively. One-on-one; one brain to one brain.

Every brain is different. No one size fits all. No group teaching situation fits all. No one tutoring process fits all. When you think about it, why should they?

For thirty-six years in a row, I flew to Boston from Fort Lauderdale every September to deliver a lecture on "Clinical Aspects of the Upper Extremity" to the first-year class at my alma mater, Boston University's School of Medicine.[5] The lecture stressed that when God creates you, he puts the "computer" we call the brain, which controls your whole body, inside your skull. That computer gives off the "big electrical cable," which we call the spinal cord, from where the "wires" we call nerves branch out. It's a complicated setup. Each of us is so different physically, with nerves and muscles interacting and developing every which way, is it such a leap to think that the central neurological electrical circuitries we call our brains should also differ? Why should each brain be the same?

Danny, a brilliant seventeen-year-old Aspie who applied for an intern position with my media company, understood this. "Sure, people's brains are like computers," he said during our interview. "The Asperger brain is different, though. You can't change the hardware in an Aspie brain. But you *can* change the software."

So all of you caring about Aspies and cheering them on, take heart! There *is* hope. Every person's brain is unique. You can change the software. You can learn how the brain of the Aspie whom you care for so much really works. But to do so, you're going to have to open not just your heart but your mind as well to understand each Aspie's unique way of "connecting the dots."

Employing the principle that every brain is different helps Rebecca reach the students she tutors. Likewise, it has helped me to understand so much about Asperger's and thus improve my relationship with my daughter a hundredfold. Once you also get this principle, you'll do a better job of helping your Aspie—no matter what his age—maximize his potential.

And if you're an Aspie—or if you're a professional expert, such as a behavioral psychologist, psychiatrist, cognitive behavioral therapist, specially trained special education teacher, educated in and having devoted your life to Asperger's syndrome[6]—reading this, don't take offense; I'm just a formerly totally clueless parent who's now a bit less clueless. I'm so lucky to have a wonderful ESE teacher Pati Fizzano, who "gets" Asperger's and autism spectrum, and my daughter, Rebecca, a brilliant Aspie who "gets it," teaching me the ropes and contributing greatly along the way.

---

1 Discrete mathematics is the study of whole numbers and geometric structures having parts that can be counted versus analysis (the fancy name for calculus), which is concerned with mathematical representations of physically continuous structures, or abstract set theory, which deals with nonintuitive notions of infinity. Got that? Me neither.

Research in discrete math increased in the latter part of the twentieth century with the development of computers, which operate in discrete steps and store data in discrete bits. Discrete math concepts are useful in studying objects and problems in computer science, such as algorithms, programming languages, cryptography, and software development. Discrete math can be looked at as a way for computer science majors to satisfy their math requirement without dirtying their hands with much calculus, which most of them hate.

One day I asked Rebecca's tutor at Georgia Tech, a PhD candidate in discrete math, what his friends with a discrete math degree do for a living. He said that one of them was breaking al-Qaeda code for the CIA and another had just gotten a job on Wall Street making $500K a year developing algorithms for a hedge fund.

2 It's not my intention to offend the true experts who have devoted their lives to the study of Asperger's or the professions relating to such disorders. It's more that I appreciate the words of Mark Twain: "I've never let my schooling interfere with my education." That's why I'm publishing this book now; I'm afraid further schooling will muddle my current rather clear vision.

3 The autistic community coined the term *neurotypical* as a label for people who are not on the autism spectrum. The term is now used for anyone who does not have atypical neurology, i.e., anyone who does not have autism, Asperger's, dyslexia, bipolar disorder, ADD/ADHD, or other similar conditions.

4 If I'm stalled on a project, I'll call my mentor, Bernie Karcinell, who taught me to pose the question that Rebecca used: "What are we trying to accomplish here?" It can be easy to lose sight of the main goal. For instance, if we're trying to change a negative behavior to a positive one, the key is the method we use. But we might be getting nowhere because we're relying on the method that always worked for other individuals. To change this individual's behavior, another method might be better, because every brain is different.

Bernie has been my friend and mentor for nearly thirty years. He's a former partner at KPMG/Peat Marwick. He's seventy-five years old and as brilliant as ever.

5 At BUSM, my first-year anatomy teacher was Dr. Elizabeth Moyer. She was a woman ahead of her time; she took guff from no one. That year she said, "You'll probably move far away, where it's nice and warm, and forget all about us." But she challenged me to return to BU to teach. I told her someday I would. One day the next year I had a lunch appointment with Dr. Moyer. But she never showed up—she had died that morning of a pulmonary embolism. My lecture to the first-year class was how I kept my promise to her.

6 Later I'll address the change in nomenclature where the term *Asperger's* has suddenly magically disappeared! Now it's just part of the spectrum (a spectrum disorder means that there is a wide variation in how the disorder affects people). In fact, all of our brains are just part of the spectrum.

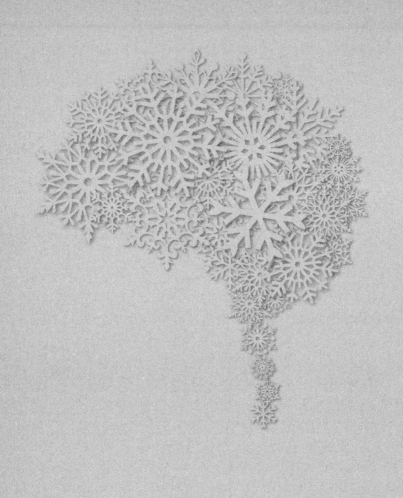

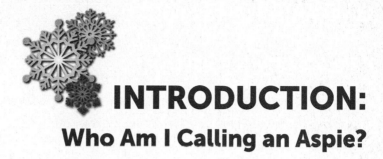

INTRODUCTION:
Who Am I Calling an Aspie?

**It ain't what they call you,
it's what you answer to.**

—*W.C. Fields*

Organizing this book was difficult for me. While I say and believe that every brain and every individual are different and unique, in the same breath I try to give chapters and characteristics names. My goal in writing this book is to give you real tools you can use in your real situation. To do that, I discovered I had to sacrifice complete uniformity, because one size does not fit all. So much of the knowledge I gained in my journey I learned from my daughter, who has Asperger's, among other issues. But the "stuff" I learned applies to all brains to varying degrees. So I call these helpful items Aspertools, real tools to help. And those people I am calling "Aspies" are not just those with Asperger's but all those with "different" brains. You'll notice that while most chapters have similar construction, I did not make the structure of each chapter 100 percent uniform across the board, because, again, one size does not fit all, and readers will use each chapter differently and to varying degrees based upon their particular situations. Generally, I organized the book this way:

- **Chapter Topic:** the main topic of concern
- **Helpful Hint:** a quick take on the issue, with a doable fix
- **Imagine You're an Aspie** (where applicable): the issue from an Aspie's point of view
- **Action Plan:** the approach to take for the situation
- **Tip from ESE Teacher Pati Fizzano:** a special insight from an expert teacher who works with "different brained" kids every day and who "gets" it
- **Thought from Rebecca Reitman:** insight from the Aspie herself, with her discrete math degree, with her brilliance, with her other issues, and with her Asperger's syndrome

Putting all these things together, I think I found the winning combination. I know you don't want long-winded explanations; you need tools you can use right now that will make a difference in your life by understanding your Aspie and helping her to live a full and maximally independent life without you.

A funny thing happened on my way to finishing this book. In May 2014, I flew to Boston for the fortieth reunion of the Boston University School of Medicine Class of 1974 (although some other years were represented). You know how at a reunion it seems like everyone asks, "So what are you up to?" It seemed even more so with me, because my career went in many different directions. In 1971, my first year of med school, I won the New England Golden Gloves heavyweight boxing championship. Then seventeen years later, as a full-time orthopedic surgeon, I turned professional heavyweight boxer and had my fifteen minutes of fame in the national media.[7]

Because of my short-lived fame, some of my classmates knew a bit about what I'd been up to. I filled them in by saying I was now involved in producing movies, documentaries, and reality TV shows, as well as writing books. When they asked what I was writing about, I'd tell them that I was finishing a book on Asperger's syndrome and different types of brains.

Invariably, the person I was talking with would launch into a story of her own and tell me about a family member who was "a bit different" but who—she'd hasten to add—"is definitely not Asperger's." I'd ask a few questions. It would quickly turn into a game of figuring out which of the book's chapters applied to her "bit different" someone.

For example, at one point a former classmate and his wife started to tell me about their daughter. The exchange went something like this:

Me: "How does your daughter do socially?"

Father: "Well, she's not really a people person. What she really loves are animals."

Me: "Where did she go to school? What did she study?"

Father: "She ended up in an agricultural school, where she studied animal husbandry."

Me: "Where is she now?"

Mother: "She lives on a ten-acre farm with a menagerie of animals. She married a man ten years older than her. She's very happy."

The word *Asperger's* didn't come up in the conversation, but it was like the proverbial elephant in the room, because people, especially parents, often run away from the stigma of a label such as Asperger's. It's a combination platter: part denial, part ignorance, part "my kid is normal," part struggle and admitting, "I don't know what to do." They feel shame/guilt/sadness. It's often easier to deny, call it something else, but there are many reasons, not the least of which is that the Aspie you care about *will* make it in the real world, and many do make it in the mainstream.

Later that evening I was introduced to an elderly couple from New Hampshire. When I told them I was a former orthopedic surgeon and had flown up from Florida, they asked how I liked retirement. I laughed and said, "Although I'm not performing surgery anymore, I'm not retired and am writing a book on Asperger's."

The man chuckled. "I'm eighty years old and not retired either. I am still practicing pediatrics."

I figured that a pediatrician with more than a half century of experience with children and teenagers might know a little about Asperger's and autism. So I asked if he had any interesting thoughts on the subject.

He said, "Back in the fifties and sixties, people didn't know what autism was. The general feeling was that whatever it was, it was caused by emotionally frigid mothers."

This led to a discussion of the PBS documentary *Refrigerator Mothers,* which chronicled the horrible ignorance of that day.[8] The elderly pediatrician's theory was that autism has always been around, but, for whatever the reason, it is much more prevalent now.

As he said this, he was gazing at the floor rather than looking me in the eye. I thought it might have something to do with his being hunched over (the orthopedist in me suspected some kind of kyphosis of his spine). But as we were ending our conversation, he said something that suggested another reason for averting my gaze. "I was always a bit different myself. Oh, they never put a label on me. But I think that today they'd probably label me as Asperger's."

There's that *L* word again: *LABELS*. Let's return to the question "Who am I calling an Aspie?" In the pages that follow, whenever I say "your Aspie," I'm referring to "that person you care about, whose different brain might be helped by some of these chapters." If the shoe fits, wear it. But forget the labels—focus on the characteristics of the individual and the tools to help her. In other words, don't view the Aspertools in this book as designed to help someone who has Asperger's; view them as designed to help an individual who has many special qualities and who *also happens* to have a few Asperger's traits, or even the whole enchilada we call Asperger's syndrome.

Don't forget: these are human beings with many endearing qualities. These "bit different" individuals might have an additional characteristic that could be "labeled" as Asperger's syndrome. But are you or am I defined in totality by a label or any one aspect of our being? No? Well, neither should Aspies.

---

7 Most people asked me how I could resolve the ethical dilemma of being a surgeon—whose mission in life is to follow the Hippocratic oath and heal people—and a boxer, who is put in the position of having to try to hurt his opponent. I started boxing when I was a kid. I won the New England Lowell Heavyweight Golden Gloves title when I was in medical school, but I turned down a $100,000 pro signing bonus that would have required that I quit school. Then seventeen years later, when Rebecca was only four years old and undergoing a risky and, at the time, experimental procedure at the Mayo Clinic, stereotactic brain surgery, I made a promise to God that if she did okay then, I'd fight the toughest guys on earth so my brain could get beat up and not hers. I finished with a pro record of thirteen wins, seven losses, and six draws. I was once ranked number twelve for about ten minutes then got killed twice on national TV. I donated all purses to children's charities, raised awareness on many children's issues, met with the president of the United States to discuss children's issues, and failed in my delusional quest to become heavyweight champion of the world.

8 From the 1950s through the 1970s, the medical establishment believed that poor mothering was the root cause of autism. Doctors presumed that the obsessive behaviors of autistic children—rigid rituals, speech difficulty, self-isolation—stemmed from their mothers' emotional frigidity. The 2002 documentary explores the legacy of blame, guilt, and self-doubt suffered by a generation of women who were branded "refrigerator mothers."

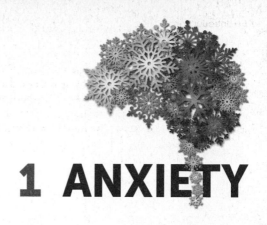

1 ANXIETY

> I am an old man and have
> known a great many troubles, but
> most of them never happened.
>
> —*Mark Twain*

> Anxiety is one little tree
> in your forest. Step back and
> look at the whole forest.
>
> —*Unknown*

Helpful Hint: Anxiety affects nearly everything an Aspie does. What makes an Aspie so anxious? The sad truth is many, many things. That's what makes it such a challenge. You must learn to recognize the signs of anxiety and then use your Aspertools to ameliorate it.

Every one of us experiences some degree of anxiety at one point or another: an overwhelming sense of apprehension and fear that often exhibits physiological symptoms. It's become so prevalent in our stressed-out society that one in five Americans now takes some kind of medication because of emotional and mental conditions that are associated with anxiety. But for Aspies, anxiety is far and away the king of the hill. Most of the actions and reactions of Aspies are related to their degree of anxiety. Once *you* realize that, you're on your way to solving many of your Aspie's problems—maybe even preventing them in the first place. Why does anxiety determine the behavior patterns of an Aspie to such a large extent? For starters, consider the following:

In the movie *Groundhog Day*, every day's events were the same as the day before, and Bill Murray's clueless newscaster character relived them over and over until he "got them right." Well, every day for Aspies is like a reverse *Groundhog Day*. The same events from the day before seem *brand new*, so each day they have to solve the same problems over and over, as if for the first time. Come to think of it, it's more like the movie *50 First Dates*, in which Drew Barrymore's character's short-term memory-loss disorder means that each night all memories of her day get erased, which severely complicates Adam Sandler's courtship of her. For Aspies, every day is a challenge as they learn how to navigate an unseen maze. Yes, it is hard to believe. That's why Aspies *love* routines and rules, as you probably have come to realize and will learn more about later in this book. I don't know why this is; some say it's poor short-term memory. I can't answer all the whys, and I do not want you to get bogged down in theories and studies. Rather, what are you going to do about it? What is the Aspie going to do about it? What's the problem? What's the solution? If there is no solution, what's the tool that can help?

Think about that. If you had to keep solving the same problems you solved the day before, if your every interaction with another human being seemed like rocket science, wouldn't you be anxious? And if you were always aware that your anxiety could escalate to a full meltdown, wouldn't that make you even more anxious?

A major source of anxiety for an Aspie is being placed in a social gathering or a new situation. Now that I'm no longer clueless about this phobia, I feel really sad when I recall all the times I lost my patience and yelled, "Stop being so stubborn!" because Rebecca wanted no part of an activity that her all-knowing father viewed as important, but which she knew would cause her great anxiety. On the occasions when I did get her to go to one of these activities, she'd want to leave almost as soon as she got there. For example, the New York Jets were scheduled to play the Miami Dolphins. I said, "Come on, Rebecca, let's go to the football game. Your favorite team, the Jets, is in town. You'll have a great time!" She was hesitant, but I coerced her to go and was nevertheless perplexed at her negative reaction once we got there. I didn't realize that the noise, the drunken fans, the bright lights on the scoreboard were an overload of stimuli for her. Looking back on it now, I feel terribly guilty at my ignorance.

Even when she is having a good time, like at a party at our house with family and friends, it's often still too taxing for her and she'll want to leave.

Imagine you're an Aspie. A big family event is coming up. You're already apprehensive, knowing the effort you'll have to exert trying to figure out what's going on, attempting to read all the nonverbal social cues, looking foolish at taking a joke literally, trying not to embarrass yourself in front of your parents and your relatives. Just thinking about it is making your anxiety levels skyrocket. You know you're going to have to fake your way through it and that it's going to be an emotionally exhausting day. Wait a minute. Maybe you can still get out of it somehow. Maybe you can come down with a fever the night before. But you know how your parents will react. You can see in your mind's eye the disappointment and even anger on their faces if you try to get out of it.

Aspies try to hide their anxiety. They bluff, they smile, they try to please you as they navigate the turbulent waters of social interaction; attempting to follow instructions; straining to interpret visual and verbal cues; doing their best to tune out interruptive sounds, smells, lights, touches. Eventually they learn to do a pretty good job of concealing it.

But take a good look at their body language. Those nervous hand motions they try to hide. That plastered-on smile. And if you look really close, those beads of sweat that sometimes form on their upper lips. Despite all these little giveaways, they still manage to hide their anxiety from their parents and other so-called neurotypicals. Why are we so easy to fool? Because we want to believe that everything's fine. Because we don't understand how our Aspie might be a genius in advanced math and yet take idioms literally, be nervous about going to a family get-together, have no common sense, or not be able to understand the simplest thing.

Action Plan: *Learn how to recognize the telltale signs of your Aspie's anxiety.* If you can learn to anticipate rising anxiety levels, you'll be able to calm him down by using Aspertools. One of the most important Aspertools is *preparation.*[9] That upcoming family event your Aspie is dreading so much? Many Aspies do just fine once they're put into a group social situation—it's getting them there that's the problem. So rather than snarl, "You're going and that's that!" try to ease their apprehension. A little encouragement goes a long way. Calculated preparation goes even further. Review who'll be there. Recall some of your Aspie's past experiences with Uncle Frank, Aunt Doris, and cousins David and Liza. Comfort him with a smile and a hug. Give him a good idea of what to expect at the function—Aspies don't like being surprised.

Aspies get anxious learning how to handle themselves in any situation and solving any problem—even ones they've solved before—as if they're learning to solve it for the first time. But they *can* learn. They *can* get better at all this. They the choice of whether to take part in a social event, their answer will always be no. *Preparation for any social event or situation is critical.* Do your best to give them the tools they need so they'll want to say yes.

---

9 In case you're wondering about medications for relieving anxiety, the jury is still out. Meds are not an end-all and be-all; on the other hand, it makes no sense to rule out all use of anti-anxiety meds. This has become a controversial area of the neurosciences.

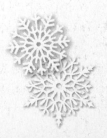

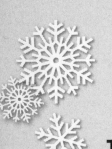

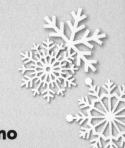

Tip from ESE Teacher Pati Fizzano

All children in school settings have some form of anxiety, even if for some it's only occasional. When Aspie students become anxious, their signs of anxiety become more noticeable through their body language, increased repetitive behavior, angry outbursts, or total avoidance of their surroundings. The anxiety may also manifest itself as a somatic complaint, such as a headache or stomach pains.

ESE teachers need to put on their detective hats to figure out why the anxiety occurred. Was it purely a behavior problem, or was it caused by sensory issues? To determine the cause, an ESE teacher will ask the Aspie if he knows what the trigger was. The teacher may speak to those who were around the Aspie, including other teachers and administrators, to get a picture of what the environment was like before the anxiety occurred. We are always trying to find ways for Aspies to cope with their anxiety and change it to avoid a recurrence.

Thought from Rebecca Reitman

Aspies are always experiencing more anxiety than they show. Even if no signs of anxiety are evident, it is present. Once we were going to my personal trainer's gym to work out. I was focused on that—getting there—but my dad wanted to have a conversation and discuss things. I just wanted a transition time between what

I was doing and where I was going and not have to fill that space with conversation.

Anxiety can be caused by placing an Aspie in a social gathering or any new situation. Having someone as my coach has helped reduce my anxiety and stress levels—it's good to have someone to talk to who truly understands my feelings. And my relationship with my parents has gotten stronger because my coach has helped them better understand the way my brain works.

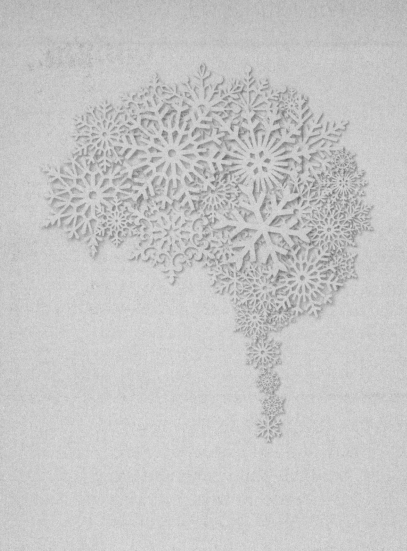

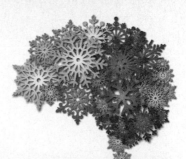

2 HYPERSENSES: SENSES ON STEROIDS

Every second of every day,
our senses bring in way too much
data than we can possibly
process in our brains.

—Peter Diamandis

Helpful Hint: You cannot understand your Aspie's
behavior and anxieties unless you take her hypersensitivity into
consideration. Each one of her five senses—sight, hearing, smell,
taste, and touch—is "on steroids." Processing all that sensory
stimuli can overload her system, and like a computer with too little
RAM to run certain applications, that overload results in a crash.

A friend of mine confessed he'd only recently discovered that his college-age son, David, had Asperger's, but he added that he'd learned much about living with the disability over the previous six months. I asked him what the single biggest change was in what he did for his son.

"Minimize loud noises in his environment. We do everything we can to keep our house nice and quiet," he replied.

I nodded. His reply brought into focus what I had just recently learned. I'm a naturally gregarious person, and I was talking a bit louder than necessary, trying to make a point to Rebecca. She put her hands over her ears and said, "Stop it!"

"That is very rude," I responded, thinking she didn't want to hear what I had to say.

Then she explained that it literally hurt her ears when I was so loud. She had no ill intent whatsoever. Up until that point, I had thought she just didn't like what I was saying. I did not realize that loud noises were to her Asperger's ears and brain what bright flashing lights were to her brain and seizure disorder. She still has to remind me about not speaking in such a loud voice, which I probably use because it is second nature to me and I don't even realize that I'm speaking so loudly. Then I thought how loud noise involves just one sense: hearing. For many Aspies, *all five* of their senses are *hypersensitive*.

This is one of the many things I wish I had known when Rebecca was growing up. Like when she would not want to be with a classmate who wore a lot of perfume and we thought it was just an excuse. I didn't realize that to her the scent of the perfume was overwhelming and nearly asphyxiating.

I thought she was overreacting when I attempted to get her to try a spicy food that she wanted no part of. Even something mild on the chili hotness scale would seem scalding hot to her.

I did not get why she used to enjoy going to a baseball game—after she got used to it—but she could never handle a loud, blaring, football game. By the time I figured all of this out, Rebecca was well into adulthood.

Principle: Your Aspie's hypersensitivity is a key source of their anxiety. LOOK AT THE DIFFERENCE BETWEEN THIS SENTENCE IN ALL CAPITAL LETTERS AND THE ONE JUST BEFORE IT IN REGULAR UPPER- AND LOWERCASE. USING ALL CAPITAL LETTERS IN TEXT IS CONSIDERED SCREAMING IN PRINT, SO WE DON'T USE THEM IN A BOOK. BECAUSE IT IS SO JARRING AND ANNOYING, IT IS HARD TO CONCENTRATE ON WHAT YOU ARE READING. This is what an Aspie feels all the time. Aspies can be driven over the edge by bangs, loud noises, the sound of chalk on a blackboard (which sounds to them like screeching), bright flashing lights, pungent aromas, awful smells, someone grabbing their arms with no warning, even funny-tasting foods.

For many Aspies, their most sensitive sense is *smell*. Experienced teachers in charge of Aspies know this and will not use any candles or room sprays in their classrooms, nor will they wear perfumes or colognes. The middle school where Rebecca teaches with Pati Fizzano has thirty students with Asperger's out of a total enrollment of 1,200. One day one of the special education teachers decided to microwave a pungent plate of food. At least half of the Aspie students became physically sick from the odor!

Another time a teacher inadvertently burned a piece of toast. She quickly resolved the problem by emptying out the charred piece of bread and all the crumbs from the toaster, then took the trash outside. Thirty minutes later, an Aspie student came into the classroom and got physically sick from the smell that by this time was barely noticeable to anyone else.

Most people like the smell of fresh popcorn, but, according to Pati, some students find it overwhelming and get sick. This isn't the case with everyone, and it might not be true of your Aspie, but, as you will learn, you will need to put your own observation skills to the test for yourself and your particular situation.

No one size fits all, and each Aspie is different; some use soothing scents to relax themselves.

(Reminder: When I use the term *Aspie*, I am not necessarily referring to the "classic Asperger's syndrome" individual; I may be referring to your Aspie, an individual who exhibits some of these traits and whose brain is a bit different from that of the "neurotypical," and that Aspie trait may very well be in you. We are all Aspies to some extent. Don't get caught up in labels. The goal is to use the Aspertools that pertain to the individual you focus on.)

Imagine you're an Aspie. You're in your room, contentedly tapping on your keyboard, listening to the soft music coming through your earphones. Without warning someone pulls off the earphones and yells, "You'd better clean this pigsty up right now!" It's your mom. Having your earphones yanked off, your mom yelling at you . . . it's too much for your brain to handle.

You're at a family event and you see your Uncle Dave approaching. You like him, but the two of you are not especially close. You're expecting him to greet you by shaking hands. Instead, he suddenly gives you a bear hug. He's squeezing you and the pressure on your skin is unbearable. This triggers an anxiety attack—the last thing you want today, in front of all your relatives.

You're used to the scent of the Mennen Skin Bracer aftershave your dad usually puts on. But today as he goes off to work and gives you a hug good-bye, he smells totally different. He's put on a different aftershave! The strange new smell confuses you. You wonder why your dad would make a major change like that without consulting you first.

You're watching TV in the dimly lit living room, lying on the couch in sweatpants and a T-shirt. You couldn't be more comfortable. Suddenly the bright overhead lights flash on. Your roommate starts barking at you to get dressed because he wants you to meet some people. Your hands start to spasm.

Action Plan: Sudden or strong stimuli of any kind are a problem for Aspies. Aside from initially startling them, the magnitude of the sensory input overloads their brain circuitry; their brains can't process it all, and they go on tilt. It's your job to be the guardian of their environments and minimize loud noises, flashing lights, strange new smells, sudden touching or grabbing, maybe even foods with strong or unusual tastes. But foremost, be calm and gentle, and talk softly.

Preparation is your key tool for dealing with sensory overload.

A poster of Muhammad Ali hanging in the boxing gym reads: THE FIGHT IS WON AND LOST WELL BEFORE THE NIGHT OF THE FIGHT. IT IS WON AND LOST IN THE GYM WITH THE WEEKS OF PREPARATION FOR THE FIGHT. Preparing Aspies for first-time experiences where their senses will be on overload can be helpful. Aspies should be given a preview of what their first ride on a train or a subway will be like. The same goes for their first visit to a baseball or football game, their first concert, even their first visit to a bakery. We can't control the world we live in, but we can prepare for that world and its experiences.

As your Aspie gets older, she will have to learn to deal with strong stimuli on her own.

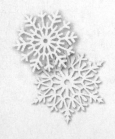

Tip from ESE Teacher Pati Fizzano

ESE teachers need to be cognizant of each Aspie student's sensory needs and limits. Each Aspie is different, and as teachers we need to help them be in control of their surroundings.

Last year I taught an ESY (extended school year) summer program at a local elementary school. Prior to meeting the students, I read all their Individual Education Plans (IEPs)[10] to get a better understanding of their needs. The IEP of one third grader, Harry, noted that he hated loud noises. I knew the school was planning a fire drill. Prior to the drill I spoke to Harry about it and gave him a set of headphones to help him deal with loud noises. The day of the drill Harry put them on in advance, and when the alarm went off, he calmly walked outside with the other students to their assigned area. An Aspertool had provided him with a lifelong coping skill.

Another student, Chrissy, was uncomfortable with taking showers because she did not like the sensation of water hitting her eyes. I suggested she try wearing swimming goggles while showering. Because of this Aspertool, Chrissy now enjoys taking a shower.

---

10 Individualized Education Program, a plan or program developed to ensure that a child who has a disability identified under the law and is attending an elementary or secondary educational institution, receives specialized instruction or services.

The weekly yoga instructor in our Social Personal class believes that the scent of lavender soothes the mind. She gives each student a cotton ball with a drop of lavender oil on it and tells them to keep it in their backpacks. If students begin feeling stress, they take the cotton ball out of their backpacks and sniff it. Another nice little Aspertool.

Teachers frequently use food to reward students for a job well done, such as popcorn or pizza. But what might be a reward for some students may trigger a negative response in an Aspie for whom that food's aroma might be too intense or overpowering. A teacher needs to be aware of what might trigger a negative response in any student.

Thought from Rebecca Reitman

I know my sensory limits. I avoid very bright lights, and I know not to look at blinking lights. I have a plethora of problems with light, such as going from light to dark or vice versa. I automatically close my eyes or look down when I transition. Ceiling fans are also a different problem because of my seizure disorder and migraines. Scented products really bother my olfactory sense, so I make it a point not to buy any fragrance items. Since I don't like wearing headphones, I avoid loud sounds by either walking away from them or leaving the room.

Each Aspie has different criteria for what they do or don't eat. For some it may be the texture of food. I am guided more by eating what is good for my stomach and avoiding what might upset it. I'm a pretty basic eater. I don't try many new foods; I'm content to stick to familiar foods that I know I like the taste.

Non-Aspies do not realize how many senses are involved in every situation. And the more senses involved in a situation, the greater the anxiety for an Aspie. For example, most of the congregants at our synagogue like it when a musician accompanies the service. But a musical instrument can interfere with my hearing the prayers. On the nights that a musician is playing in the background, I don't attend services. When Aspies' brains have to process too many stimuli, they can't focus.

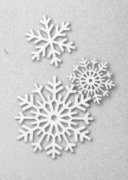

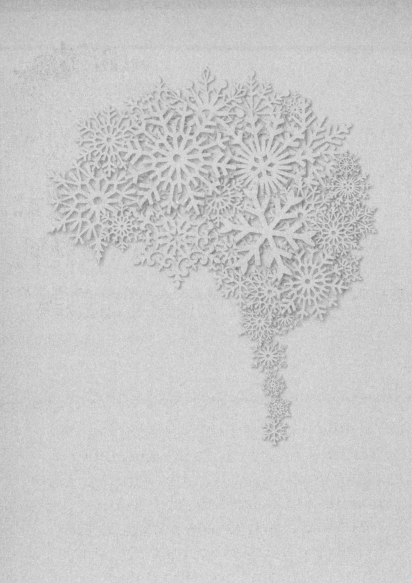

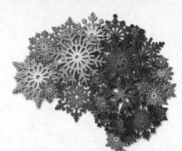

3 OBSERVATION: "ELEMENTARY, MY DEAR WATSON"

The common eye sees only the outside of things, and judges by that, but the seeing eye pierces through and reads the heart and the soul, finding there capacities which the outside didn't indicate or promise, and which the other kind couldn't detect.

—*Mark Twain*

You see, but you do not observe.

—*Sherlock Holmes*

Helpful Hint: Carefully observing your Aspie's behavior can be one of your most effective tools for helping him. Put on your Sherlock Holmes detective cap and observe. This is particularly important if you are to help the Aspie keep his anxiety from getting out of hand. Look, listen, sense, learn. Open your eyes and ears as you do your heart.

I offered this same advice recently to a mom I'd met at a charity fundraising event. Her twenty-year-old son, a college student, had just moved back home. She was upset because he seemed to be languishing. I asked what his interests were. Mom didn't have a clue. I asked what he was studying in school, still trying to get a handle on what he was passionate about. She replied, "We are forcing him to go to college. He doesn't want to go."

After I explained the Sherlock Holmes and observation theory, I saw the lightbulb go off in her head as she blurted, "You're my savior!"

No, I'm not. I'm just here to say that with a little understanding and patience, we can help nurture brains that are just a little bit different, and often very misunderstood, to achieve success.

I n Sir Arthur Conan Doyle's timeless stories about Sherlock Holmes, the greatest fictional detective of all time, Dr. Watson would frequently tell Holmes how brilliant he was. Holmes would brush aside the compliment by telling his sidekick that all he did was observe.

"A Scandal in Bohemia" begins with Holmes receiving a visit from Watson, whom he has not seen for two months.[11]

Holmes notices details about his friend and quickly deduces nearly everything Watson has done for the past eight weeks. After Holmes explains to the astonished doctor how he made these deductions, Watson says it seems so logical that he should be able to do it himself. After all, his eyesight is as good as his friend's.

Holmes replies, "You see, but you do not observe. . . . For example, you have frequently seen the steps which lead up from the hall to this room?"

Watson says he has climbed the stairs hundreds of times. Holmes asks how many steps there are. When Watson says he doesn't know, Holmes says, "Quite so! You have not observed. And yet you have seen. . . . Now, I know that there are seventeen steps, because I have both seen and observed."

So open your eyes and start observing your Aspie, in proper Holmesian fashion, for signs of anxiety, sensory overload, and other issues. As the great detective might say, you need to do more than simply see; you need to study him and observe.

Let me tell you a story that underscores the distinction between simply seeing and diligent observation. Several years ago I wrote, directed, and produced the full-length movie *The Square Root of 2*, which was fiction inspired by the true story of a young woman with learning disabilities fighting an unfair higher educational system. The woman who inspired the story was my daughter, Rebecca, in the movie played by Darby Stanchfield (you may know her as Abby Whelan on the TV show *Scandal*), who is not only a very talented actress but also a highly observant one. In preparation for the filming of *The Square Root of 2*, she never stopped studying Rebecca. And in the movie, in addition to the many nuances she practiced, she exhibits some of Rebecca's repetitive hand motions.

For years I had thought that my daughter's repetitive, idiosyncratic hand motions had a neurological basis. After all, Rebecca has twenty-three vascular brain tumors and has had two major brain surgeries, although you'd never guess this from talking to her.[12] Not until a few years later did I learn of Rebecca's Asperger's, the role that anxiety plays for most Aspies, and the things that produce anxiety in her. I now know that her hand motions are a sign of anxiety. When we're together, I look for those signs of anxiety, try to figure out what is adding to her stress and anxiety levels, and then try to help defuse the situation. Back then I didn't know to do that. Now I do.

Many scenes in *The Square Root of 2* in general illustrate classic Aspie scenarios, which I did not realize at the time of production. Darby Stanchfield's amazing, nuanced portrayal of an Aspie occurred despite the ignorance of this clueless dad filmmaker. Why? Because Darby studied and observed Rebecca directly.

Action Plan: You can't solve a problem if you don't recognize the problem's manifestations. *Studied observation should be one of the key tools in your Asperger's toolkit.* Use it to watch for the symptoms of anxiety, or for indications that the Aspie's hypersenses are being forced to process too many stimuli, or to determine which rewards to use to reinforce positive behavior, or to recognize signs that your Aspie is being overwhelmed. Being overwhelmed leads to the cataclysm we're about to encounter— the meltdown.

11 In the timeline assembled by Sherlock Holmes scholar Brad Keefauver, "A Scandal in Bohemia" transpires in March 1888, some two and a half months after the previous Holmes adventure, "The Valley of Fear." It is during this interval that Watson gets married and goes on a honeymoon.

12 I'll never forget the intense experience of the surgery waiting room at the Mayo Clinic in Minnesota, praying and making every kind of deal with God I could, as Rebecca underwent the pioneering stereotactic surgery that saved her life against great odds. As part of that deal, I returned to boxing at age thirty-seven and ultimately to the ten-round, main event, professional heavyweight boxing ranks, donating my purses to children's charities . . . while continuing to practice orthopedic surgery. But that's a story for another day.

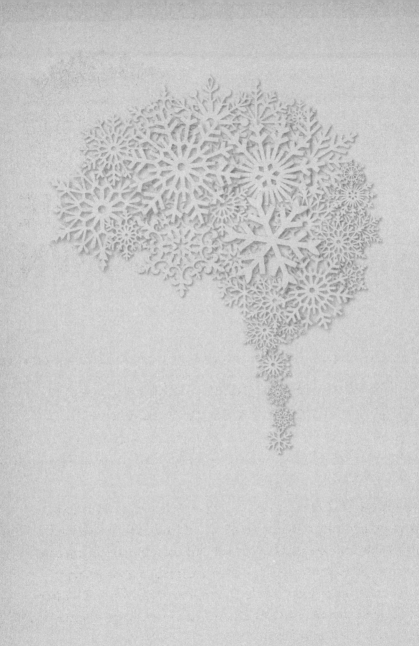

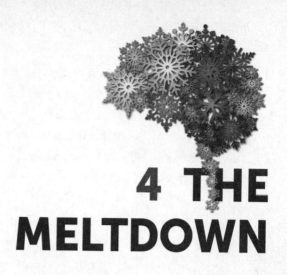

4 THE MELTDOWN

Sometimes it takes a
meltdown to cool down.

—*Evinda Lepins, author of* Back to Single

Helpful Hint: It's critical to find ways to defuse an oncoming Aspie meltdown, because once it's underway, there's nothing the Aspie can do except ride it out. And there's nothing you can do except provide quiet support in a safe place. By learning to recognize the triggers that lead up to the meltdown, you'll often be able to ease the situation. Here is where an ounce of prevention is truly worth a ton of cure.

Principle: When marathon runners "hit the wall" and can't go a single step farther, it's not just due to physical factors like cramping and blisters. Psychological and neurological issues come into play as well. They just can't do it. It's the same with an Aspie meltdown. This force of nature—akin to a volcanic eruption—is a similar confluence of neurological, psychological, and physical factors.

For an Aspie, a meltdown and a temper tantrum are two entirely different things. The tantrum is about manipulation. For instance, a young Aspie may scream, "I want a puppy!" over and over. As a parent, you do your best to ignore it, but they won't give up. They'll demand a puppy until you give in (which you should not do) or until they get tired. You have to teach them that rather than throw a tantrum, they should use logic and rational persuasion to win you over to their point of view. (Yes, this can be taught with time and effort, and with rules, rewards, and consequences.)

But when Aspies have a meltdown, they're not begging for anything. Rebecca said that what might start out as an issue that is unreasonable to the Aspie, is then acted upon and seen by others as a "tantrum," and after this the meltdown starts. For example, one time Rebecca's work schedule was changed without first consulting her. It was final; there was no going back, so she had to surrender to it. Rebecca saw this as deception because Pati had told her one thing but then changed it. Pati wanted to talk about what had already been established and that this was the way it had to be. Rebecca was furious, calling Pati a liar. She kept repeating that there was nothing to talk about and got increasingly anxious until she had a meltdown. Finally, she just left, knowing that it is better to remove yourself from the situation to a safe place. A meltdown is an Aspie crying out in anguish for someone to get her to a safe, quiet place, and either leave her alone or quietly comfort her. She's overwhelmed in every way a human being can be overwhelmed.

An Asperger's meltdown can be compared to an epileptic seizure. Simplistically speaking, in the case of epilepsy,[13] the brain undergoes hyperactive electrical sensitivity, which can trigger a seizure. For someone with epilepsy, blinking or flashing lights can trigger a seizure. For those with Asperger's syndrome, the equivalent of flashing lights can be someone invading their personal space or suddenly putting her hands on them, a strong scent, a loud noise, a funny taste, or merely something unexpected. Aspies will tell you that a meltdown can be the result of one of these triggers or an accumulation of them. (Plus, many Aspies have other neurological and psychological components that overlap.)

Every Aspie has a different description of what a meltdown feels like. One says that when the pressure builds inside her, it's like the cartoon character with steam coming out its ears before its head explodes, but Aspies all agree on one thing: once a meltdown begins, there's nothing they can do until it runs its course.

Consequently, meltdowns, like seizures, should be avoided at all costs. Meltdowns can have dire consequences for an Aspie, such as being physically harmed, getting arrested, being incarcerated—or something far worse.

If you don't recognize the situation in time to defuse it, this can feel like a parent's worst nightmare. You may be tempted to ask God, "Why are you doing this to *me*?" and scream at the Aspie, "Knock it off! Get used to the real world!" This is about the worst thing you can do. You must be able to recognize the telltale signs of when the Aspie is experiencing stimuli or events that, left unchecked, will lead to a meltdown. Don't be afraid to make a mountain out of a molehill. If you use *observation* to see these signs, and take preventive action, the molehill won't become a mountain.

Action Plan: Use *observation* to identify all the triggers that can set off your Aspie. If you want to keep track of them and maybe share them with other caring third parties, write them down in a *journal*. A journal can help you put the pieces of the puzzle together. Once you learn all the signs of mounting anxiety, you should be able to defuse the situation. If the situation is beyond defusing, your only option is to hustle the Aspie off to her safe place (which we'll learn more about in the next chapter).

As your Aspie gets older, she will have to learn to manage defusing the meltdown without you through self-soothing or personal prevention methods. The goal is to become independent as much as possible. If she feels her anxiety rising and a meltdown approaching, she will know what to do next. She will find her safe place, take an action that begins to reduce her anxiety (such as pacing back and forth), think of what made her anxiety levels rise, and then engage in an interest (such as drawing) to help her forget about her anxiety.

Professionals, such as psychologists, and others specifically trained in this area—for example, yoga instructors—can teach Aspies methods for defusing the meltdown themselves. Not everyone can afford a psychologist or a coach, but every Aspie should have someone they can talk to.

---

13 I believe there's a higher incidence of epilepsy in autism and Asperger's syndrome individuals than in the general population, and the same goes for other psychological and neurological syndromes. There's overlap between these neurological and psychological syndromes. That's why psychiatrists have to pass the neurology boards and neurologists have to pass the psychiatry boards.

Tip from ESE Teacher Pati Fizzano

If a student is going through a meltdown, the attitude of the ESE teacher or whoever is with that student (it could be anyone from the assistant principal to a cafeteria worker) is critical. They should not overreact. The best thing to do is to take the student to a calming place. (In our school we take them to an indoor garden.) The teacher needs to remain positive and do whatever it takes to calm down the student. Comfort the student; let her know you're there for her. An ESE teacher may end up sitting on the floor, because you want the student looking at you, and so you should be at her eye level. Offering a gentle touch can help.

Every situation is different. Some want to be left alone. Others don't mind being handled, but only in a certain way. For instance, some like hugs. Others like having their backs gently rubbed, but you can't get near their hands. This is more of an art than a science. It's always best to ask the Aspie how to deal with it.

Once we see that the meltdown is over, we walk the student back to class. We don't want a meltdown to be a drawn-out process or something used as an avoidance technique.

Some children will show signs of a meltdown beginning. For example, their faces turn red, their eyes will become deep, and they may even pace. Once the meltdown begins, they may start screaming, kicking, and hitting. They may even try to cause harm to themselves because they are so frustrated about losing control.

I have one student who has high anxiety. He is very smart and is a straight-A student in all advanced classes. However, if the teacher says, "Pop quiz," he will go into an extreme meltdown that takes him at least twenty minutes to recover from. We teach the children strategies to help them cope with these triggers to circumvent the meltdown. For this student I told him that when the teacher says, "Pop quiz," he should keep his pencil down, take five deep breaths, look over the quiz, and *then* begin. This works for him.

I never punish a student for having a meltdown. Meltdowns are part of the Aspie world. I don't want them to harm themselves, so I devise positive strategies to help them. For example, one of my students in elementary school would throw his chair, desk, and even books constantly during a meltdown. I read over his report and knew of his history. When I met him for the first time, I sat down and explained to him that his behavior is unacceptable for middle school and gave him rules. For example: "During a meltdown, use a safe pass and walk to the garden. If you throw anything during a meltdown, you will get a FINE." (The fine is points off an auction in which the students can participate at the end of the year). Twelve weeks into our school year, this student had not thrown one thing and follows the rules about meltdowns.

I feel that once you have rules, rewards, and consequences, the Aspies will deliver. Parents need to know that they cannot get frustrated with the child's meltdowns; it's a part of her life.

Thought from Rebecca Reitman

I never really knew what a meltdown was until decades later, long after I'd moved out of my parents' house. Since my dad did not understand at the time, he would react by yelling more at me, which shut me down while concurrently causing anger and fear. When an Aspie is going through a meltdown, let her take the wave and just stay out of the way.

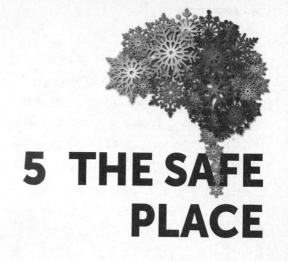

5 THE SAFE PLACE

There's nothing I like better than going to my apartment, closing the door, cooking my little dinner for one and just tuning out. My apartment really is my haven. It's a nest where I go to heal.

—*Tim Gunn*

For Mickey Mantle, the Yankees' locker room was a sanctuary, a safe haven where he was understood, accepted and, when necessary, exonerated.

—*Jane Leavy*, The Last Boy: Mickey Mantle and the End of America's Childhood

Helpful Hint: Everyone in this crazy frenetic world at some point needs an escape route to a safe place where they can have a time-out. But no one needs it more than an Aspie. Make sure Aspies know they have a safe place, a refuge where they can go to do an emotional "reboot." That knowledge is their safety valve, and knowing that there's a pathway to that safe place is their security blanket.

O ur brains are like a computer: they need to reboot now and then. For those of us who are fortunate enough to be sound sleepers, this reboot occurs at night. Even so, our brains sometimes need a time-out during the day as well. But the Aspie brain may need several such daytime time-outs.

Aspies need a safe place to have a time-out. They also need to *know* they have that safe place and that it's easy for them to get to. In the home, that might mean escaping to their bedrooms. In a school or work setting, it might mean finding a room not in use. In a car, about the only thing you can do is to provide silence, or let them put on their earbuds.

Imagine you're an Aspie. You feel your anxiety rising and a meltdown approaching. But from experience, you know what to do next.

1) Find your safe place (your apartment).
2) Pace back and forth (you're not sure why, but this begins to reduce your anxiety).
3) Think of what happened to make your anxiety levels rise.
4) Engage in your obsession or hyper-interest (drawing, singing, reading a comic book, whatever it is), because you know if you do this, you will forget about your anxiety and begin to feel better.

Principle: When the pressure is mounting, when stimuli are coming at us so fast and furious that we can't process them all, we all need a release or a place to go where we can practice a relaxation technique. All children—and even adults—need a safe and peaceful refuge where they can take a timeout when they need one. Even Superman had his Fortress of Solitude. Maybe beneath that superhero costume he was an Aspie.

That thought has occurred to others. For instance, in a blog titled "Superman Is an Aspie," writer Mame Zirro notes that in the movie *Man of Steel,* nine-year-old Clark Kent is at school, being overwhelmed by all the incoming stimuli he perceives with his super-senses: lights, movement, scratching, clock ticking, voices, feelings and sights beyond what humans normally see. He falls to the floor. The school calls his mother, Martha Kent. Later, Martha talks with Clark and asks him what's bothering him.

> Clark: *The world's too big, Mom.*
> Martha: *Then make it small. Focus on my voice. Pretend it's an island out in the ocean. Can you see it?*
> Clark: *I see it . . .*

Watching the movie, Zirro's eleven-year-old son, whom she suspects has Asperger's, told her, "That's what it's like for me. Well, not exactly, because I don't have x-ray vision. But it's like everything is coming at me."[14]

In the case of Aspies, it's important that the appropriate specialist, such as a psychologist, psychiatrist, yoga instructor, music therapist, etc., teach them how to develop their own relaxation techniques, even if it's just putting a headset on and listening to soothing music. Having their personal relaxation techniques will maximize Aspies' independence.

Action Plan: Ensure that your Aspie has a safe place for a time-out, that he knows there's "a safe place," and that the safe place is easy to get to. In the home, that might mean escaping to his bedroom. In a school or work setting, it might mean finding a safe place such as a room not in use. In a car, there's no place to retreat to, and it may be that the only thing you can do is to provide silence. Or let him put on earbuds. Quiet comfort.

---

14 http://writemybrainsout.wordpress.com/2014/01/16/superman-has-aspergers/

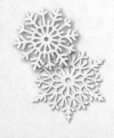

Tip from ESE Teacher Pati Fizzano

At the beginning of the semester, the school issues a Safe Pass to all of our Asperger's students. The Safe Pass allows the students, at any time, to go to their safe place, which at our school is an indoor garden. The pass is their security blanket.

Use of the pass is monitored to ensure that students do not abuse it or use it as an avoidance technique. If they abuse it, they lose it! When I issue the pass, I role-play a scenario to demonstrate the consequences of having it taken away. I often tell the story of two former students, Mary and Rocky.

Mary seldom used her pass, but during her few anxiety attacks, the pass allowed her to leave the classroom and go to the indoor garden. I'd go with her and talk with her. When she felt better, I'd escort her back to class.

Rocky was different. He hated math and all he wanted to do was play video games on his phone. Whenever he used his pass and I met up with him in the indoor garden, he never showed any anxiety. He always seemed fine.

I began tracking Rocky's Safe Pass usage and saw a pattern. It seemed that every time he was facing a math test, he used his pass as an avoidance technique. As a consequence, he lost the use of his pass. A month later Rocky started to panic during a math test. Because of his past behavior, his teacher thought he was faking it.[15] It was like the boy who cried wolf. If Rocky had still had his pass, he could have used it to go to the garden. Instead, he ended up having an extreme meltdown.

After listening to the two scenarios, all the students chose to be like Mary.

Thought from Rebecca Reitman

Aspies need to know they have a safe place and an escape route to get there. When I feel overwhelmed, the place I feel most safe and secure is my own apartment. When I'm tutoring, my safe place is Pati's home. These are the two places I feel the most comfortable.

Having the escape route is vital. If family get-togethers or other events start to overwhelm Aspies, they need to be able to say it's time to go. If they don't drive, they need to have someone who is willing to transport them home. Feeling like they're being held hostage will in and of itself make an Aspie's anxiety level soar.

---

15 It takes practice for the teachers to understand when a child with Asperger's is about to have a meltdown. They need to understand each and every child, which is difficult when you have about 110 students each day. This is why case managers, like me, are so important to the students.

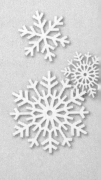

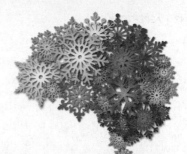

6 RUDENESS, TRUTH TELLING, AND MANNERS

You can be strong
and true to yourself without
being loud and rude.

—*Paula Radcliffe, English long-distance runner*

Helpful Hint: Aspies must learn that rudeness is unacceptable, and that being rude will incur consequences. They may need an explanation of why their act was rude.

Principle: Deliberate rudeness on the part of the Aspie is unacceptable. Yet accuse an Aspie of being rude and her first line of defense will be, "But I was just telling the truth." I thought of this when I saw the movie *August: Osage County*. Whenever Violet Weston, portrayed by Meryl Streep, said something mean-spirited and was called on it, she'd say, "I'm just truth telling. Some people are antagonized by the truth." The Aspie must be shown how the truth can be told kindly and politely, without rudeness. Also, Aspies must understand that they must have good manners and acceptable behavior, even if they perceive that their personal space is being invaded, or if their extreme territoriality of property is accidentally violated.

People often don't want to hear the truth, particularly at an inopportune time. A thin line separates the rudeness of telling a truth that inadvertently hurts another's feelings from pure rudeness. Nevertheless, hurting another's feelings by telling the truth and speaking in a nasty tone, as well as saying unpleasant things, are both examples of rude behavior, and neither one is acceptable. But Aspies are prone to engaging in the truth-telling type of rudeness.

Let me give you an example. In the after-school program at the middle school where they work, Rebecca and Pati tutor a fifth grader named Tony. When they assigned Tony to write about the most important person or thing to him, Tony chose his computer. Pati tried to persuade him that his mother, who was fighting cancer, might be a more appropriate subject. But Tony maintained that his computer was more important to him than his mom.

Pati winked at Rebecca and, presuming her to be an ally, asked what she thought Tony should do. But Rebecca fell back on her own Aspie trait of telling the truth (which, in this case, she did not consider rude) and took Tony's side.

Tony's choice of subject matter got back to his mother, who was understandably hurt. Pati explained to her that she couldn't make Tony write what he didn't feel. To Tony (and many Aspies), the computer *is* more important than a parent—it's always there, it never yells at him, and he can communicate with it more easily than with his parents, without all the stress. It's the truth, and the truth hurts, especially to an Aspie's parent. Tony's choice of a subject was typically Aspie.

Rebecca doesn't always take Tony's side. She often gets frustrated with him and vice versa. She wants to teach kids who want to learn and loses patience trying to help those who don't seem to care about that. Tony, like many fifth graders, wants to play after school, and this is where the two of them don't see eye to eye. Recently, Tony began another after-school program that involves physical activity. When Tony's mother—who works at our school—asked Rebecca, "Do you miss Tony?" she very honestly replied, "No, the classroom is much quieter and I can focus more on tutoring the students who want to learn." Of course, this is not what Tony's mother wanted to hear—she loves her child with all her heart and wants to hear good things about him, as all mothers want to hear about their children. Rebecca was not being rude—simply honest—and although a neurotypical might have thought the same thing, she might have said it a different way to soften the blow.

The next example illustrates the second type of rudeness: nastiness approaching full-blown aggression. Many Aspies are territorial about their personal possessions, and some react violently to another person touching them.

Joey, a full-grown Aspie, was flying home from college, accompanied by his mother. The flight was full, as was the shelf for carry-on luggage. Joey was trying to squeeze his overflowing backpack into the overhead compartment. A female flight attendant approached Joey, smiled, said, "Here, let me do that for you," and took the bag from Joey.

A neurotypical would have said, "Thank you." But the flight attendant's offer of assistance triggered rage in Joey, who thought he was under attack. He yanked the attendant's hand from his bag and yelled, "Don't touch my backpack!" His outburst alarmed the passengers and made the air marshals and flight crew suspect that the backpack might contain a bomb. Fortunately, his mother was able to defuse the situation before Joey got tackled or taken off the plane.

During the flight, she explained to Joey why his actions were not socially acceptable and how he might handle the situation if it came up again. When they got home, Joey and his mother revisited what happened and engaged in role-playing to teach Joey conflict resolution.

Action Plan: Aspies must understand that others cannot see their "disability"—there's no prosthetic limb or wheelchair to identify their disorder to strangers. The other person won't realize that they're dealing with someone who may react quite differently from what they expect.

The Aspie must be taught that there are times when telling the truth is rude and that they need to be polite in their verbal and written communications. Just because they want something, they don't have the right to be rude about it. They need to be patient with others, in the same way that neurotypicals who don't understand certain things about Aspies must be patient with them. If an Aspie is rude, make sure she understands exactly why what she did or said was rude (you may have to dissect the action or statement into understandable segments) and that the next time it happens there will be consequences. Rudeness can do more than make them disliked or alienate those who want to help them. Rudeness can get them beat up, suspended or expelled from school, or even arrested. *There must be zero tolerance for rudeness, rage, and temper tantrums.*

Training the Aspie to behave by society's rules is a challenge for everyone who plays a part in the Aspie circle: the parent, the caring third party, and the Aspies themselves. The Aspie circle is an important tool and will be discussed in further detail throughout the book.

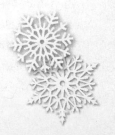

Tip from ESE Teacher Pati Fizzano

At school we have zero tolerance for bullying and rudeness. If one of my students is rude, I will say, "You're being rude." Using one-word names helps the students remember the lessons they were taught on that subject. In our curriculum we call these terms "buzzwords," which represent complex social behaviors that can be identified in a few simple words. For instance, if Rebecca starts speaking in a loud voice, I'll say, "tone." She will instantly lower the volume of her voice.

Aspies have a hard time learning manners just by watching their parents or other adults. In school we teach a range of lessons on proper etiquette through social stories. These include how to eat with utensils and not with the fingers; not chewing with your mouth open; not getting up from the dinner table while others are still eating, by employing the strategy of waiting until someone else first leaves the table; even saying "please" and "thank you." At holiday time, we suggest that students help prepare the meal instead of isolating themselves in their rooms watching TV or playing video games.

In terms of truth telling, I can't say that Aspies never lie, but I do feel they lie less than other people. When Aspies say something, it is exactly how they feel. Watch what you ask an Aspie if you can't handle the truth. This is where many people feel that Aspies are being extremely rude . . . but are they? Or is it that we can't handle their answers?

Remember that children with autism are like puzzle pieces (see the logo for AutismSpeaks.org). Each piece of the puzzle is a deficit they need to learn. I do everything possible to figure them out, understand them, learn their quirks, see what motivates them, and then teach them. This is how each of those puzzle pieces fits in. It takes time, patience, and plenty of learning and teaching, but eventually the puzzle will be completed and the rewards are endless.

Thought from Rebecca Reitman

On many occasions people have told me that my answer to a question was rude. I feel I'm being honest. If you don't want the brutal truth when you ask an Aspie a question, be patient and give them time to formulate a more polite and more politically acceptable answer. For example, an Aspie might call someone "fat," while I would say they were "thermally gifted." If I care about a person and I think that the truth of what I say will hurt them, I just won't answer.

Aspies need to know *why* something is rude. We don't master things the first time, or even the second or third time, necessarily, so be patient. If you ask a question, know that we are going to tell the truth. We probably won't be as cautious if it's about someone we don't like at the moment.

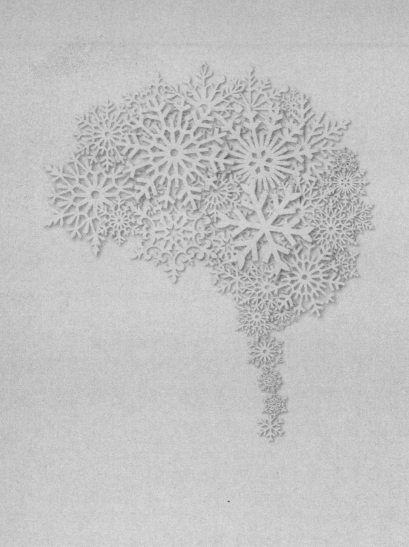

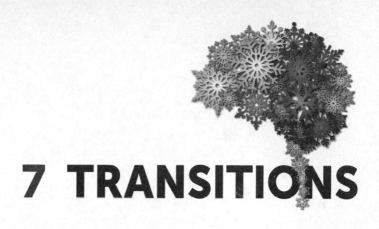

7 TRANSITIONS

> Life is pleasant. Death is peaceful.
> It's the transition that's troublesome.
>
> —Isaac Asimov

Helpful Hint: Aspies have trouble going from one activity to another or from one environment to another. You'll need to work with your Aspie to help him make the type of quick transitions required in the real world.

Principle: Aspie brains have an inertia problem—the circuitry does not allow their brains to quickly move from one scenario to another. As a result, Aspies tend to stay focused on one thing. They can't switch to a new thought process or a new activity, or register a new location or a new topic, without first taking time to prepare for the change. It's as if their brains need a mini-reboot. Add to this the fact that for many they are starting from scratch each day as they relearn the maze. Each little step can be tough for the Aspie.

Let's study this principle through a couple of examples. Going to and from class—gym class in particular—is transitional overload for many Aspies. It's the type of minor transition that neurotypicals take for granted, but because it involves many steps, it can intimidate Aspies. They have to leave their previous class, go to the locker room, change into their gym attire, go outside for the physical education activity, then come back inside, go to the locker room to change back into their school clothes, and get to the next class on time. ESE teachers who specialize in Asperger's syndrome understand how hard all these transitions are; that's why many Aspies are exempted from gym class and must get their exercise elsewhere.

Also, changing topics in the middle of a conversation, or even going from talking about one person to another, constitute the types of transitions that the Aspie brain has trouble processing. Patience is required.

Imagine you're an Aspie. Your dad is telling you how well you did at the family get-together last weekend. You're following what he's saying until he shifts gears and asks what you think about a new SUV he's considering buying. Now you're confused. Your brain is still engaged in processing the discussion of the family function and can't register this car that came out of nowhere. Wait, now your dad has started peppering you with questions about your schoolwork. Aargh! Why are conversations so difficult?

Action Plan: Whoa! Slow down! For your Aspie, conversations with others, even you, are difficult enough. If you start jumping from topic to topic, your Aspie's anxiety level will rise pretty quickly. Say, "New topic," then pause before you switch subjects. This gives the Aspie time to recalibrate. When you ask Aspies a question, be patient. Give them time to form their thoughts and put them into words. Let them finish what they're saying before you ask them a follow-up question. *Patience* is a handy tool to have in your kit of Aspertools. Ample use of it will help improve the Aspie's ability to process transitions in conversations as well as in life.

Of course, preparation is important, particularly for life's major transitions. We need to prepare Aspies for the big transitions that come into everyone's life, whether they're positive ones, like moving, getting promoted to the next grade or entering college, or changing jobs; or negative ones, such as various types of failures, an illness, or the death of a loved one.

Steady routines of positive activities in familiar surroundings are warm, fuzzy, security blankets for Aspies.

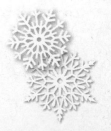

Tip from ESE Teacher Pati Fizzano

Transitions at school are tough on Aspies. In elementary school they rarely have to change classrooms, but once they get to middle school they have to change rooms up to six times a day. All this moving around makes Aspies very anxious. Many Aspies need a visual Aspertool, like a chart, to help them process all these room changes. I give them a map of the school and highlight their classes and the way to get from one class to another.

Ending a class can be another difficult transition. Aspies can't just stop what they're doing and leave the classroom, especially when they're having fun. If the students are having a lot of fun in a group activity, I know they'll need a five-minute warning to let them know they need to start cleaning up or logging off their computers. If I don't give them the alert and the bell rings, they will begin yelling and screaming. That's why they need a warning.

Also, especially with sixth graders in particular, if I see a student is overwhelmed, I allow them to leave class two minutes ahead of the bell to get a head start while the hallways are clear. Our school also allows all ASD students to leave school two minutes early to catch their buses, which has worked out very well for them.

Thought from Rebecca Reitman

A source of anxiety for many Aspies is being asked a question but not given enough time to answer. Displaying patience after you ask a question is important. Aspies can't always process things quickly. Give them time to formulate their answers.

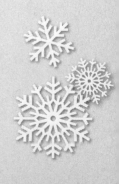

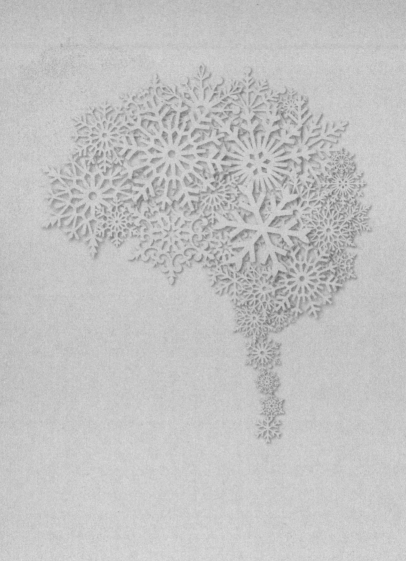

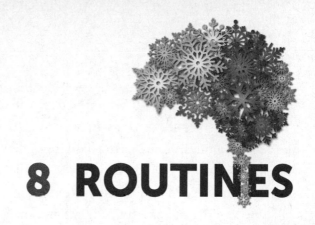

8 ROUTINES

It's a hard thing to leave any
deeply routine life, even
if you hate it.

—*John Steinbeck,* East of Eden

Helpful Hint: Aspies depend on the comfort and familiarity
of positive routines. To create a successful routine for an Aspie,
build it one step at a time; this will give the Aspie confidence in it.
If a routine that's going well needs to be altered, change it bit
by bit or in chunks rather than all at once. Since Aspies don't like
changes or surprises in their surroundings, if you see a change
coming to their environments, give them as much advance
warning as possible. The more major the change, the more
critical the preparation.

Comfort. Routine. Familiarity. Knowing where things are. Knowing how a trusted individual will act. These things give Aspies the security they need in their activities and their surroundings. Aspies have a hard time adjusting to new environments, new people, and new activities. If all five of their hypersenses get overloaded by unfamiliar stimuli and sensations, Aspies will have to do a major readjustment and may very well have a meltdown. They must greet and deal with new people. They have to learn new geography. But it overwhelms the Aspie brain. When they go someplace new and leave their familiar routines behind, it takes them a while to get comfortable.

Imagine you're an Aspie. You are preparing to face the new day, and you look forward to it because you're in a good routine. You put on your favorite sweatshirt, your most comfortable jeans, your sweat socks and sneakers, and you're set to go! Next it's your standard breakfast: a bowl of melon and strawberries, a toaster waffle smothered in butter and syrup, and a glass of milk. You love your routine: doing the same things every morning in the same order. Life is good.

Then the phone rings. Or worse, the doorbell rings. It's your parent (or friend or coach) saying the plans have changed. Your routine is suddenly changed as well. You think, "Wait a minute. Today you want me to dress up in a suit and tie? And wear black leather shoes? It's not fair. Why did you get me into that good routine in the first place if you were just going to take me out of it? I'm back at the start of the maze again. Now you're pointing at your watch and yelling at me. You don't understand how a loud voice reverberates in my head. I see

you're disappointed in me, but I don't know what
to do. All I want to do is eat my usual breakfast, but
you're saying there's no time, we'll have to grab a
quick bite at some restaurant I've never heard of. . . ."

It's not that you should never ask an Aspie to wear a suit or have a different breakfast. But you should *respect her routine if it's working*. If the routine is accomplishing its goal and it's socially acceptable in the real world, it should not be belittled or discarded. It's taken your Aspie a while to get comfortable with a routine that is helping her navigate the activities of daily living. If you're going to ask her to change that routine, you should have a good reason. You should also give advance notice, an explanation of why the routine is being changed, some encouragement, and maybe some help and preparation adapting to the new set of tasks.

If Aspies fall out of a positive routine, one with good structure and activities, or they are asked to change it, it can be difficult for them to get back into that routine or to start another positive one.

Holidays and summer breaks are challenges for Aspies because it takes them out of their school routines. During any holiday break, families should try to keep their children's routine as intact as possible by sticking with their established daily structure as best they can. They should wake up at the usual time, eat at the usual time, and go to bed at the same time. Try to keep the number of activities down to a manageable few.

If you decide to go on vacation, the Aspertool is to prepare them as much as possible so they will feel comfortable in their new surroundings. Find pictures online of where you're going and show them to your Aspie. If you're taking a cruise, show her the ship's layout ahead of time.

For an upcoming holiday party or event, parents might want to role-play with their Aspies in terms of what they'll be doing at the event, where they'll be sitting, who they'll be sitting with, even what's on the menu. Letting them know as much of this as possible will eliminate any surprises for the Aspie. (Aspies tend not to like the unexpected, so forget that surprise birthday party you were thinking about.) Plan for the possibility of an anxiety attack or meltdown (this may include bringing a sitter). But do not cancel the event, as this might upset the other children and spouses.

Even neurotypicals enjoy the comfortable routine of familiar surroundings. Remember how frustrating it was when you went to a new supermarket and couldn't find the tomato sauce? The first time I went to a Costco, I went with someone who shopped there all the time. I tagged along like a little kid, since there were no signs to indicate where anything was.[16] That day it took me forever to find everything on my list. My second trip there was only slightly more efficient.

Supermarket shopping is anything but routine for an Aspie. Try to understand why it's so overwhelming. First, Aspies must generate a shopping list. Then they have to arrange to get to the supermarket. Once there, they have to navigate that store's unique layout to find all the items on their lists, all the while battling the fluorescent lights and trying to tune out the chatter of all the customers and deal with their close proximity to the Aspie. To Aspies, a large supermarket seems like a foreign country. That's why many of them avoid food shopping altogether. If they do go to a supermarket, they need a lot of advance preparation.

Imagine you're an Aspie. You love the comfort level of routine and predictability. But today your mom has brought you with her to a new supermarket. The lighting is strange. So many colors. So many aisles. So many signs that make no sense. You don't know where anything is. The wheels of the shopping cart squeal. The fluorescent lights hum. An elderly couple is arguing over which brand of aluminum foil is a better deal. A man is talking loudly into his phone, asking someone which items he needs for dinner. Too much noise for you to focus. And while you're trying to navigate your way through the maze of food aisles while your senses are under assault, your mom shoves a shopping list in your face and starts talking to you about tonight's dinner. You might feel a little bit clumsy as you attempt to traverse the foreign surroundings.

Rebecca surprised us when she broached the subject of moving from her beautiful apartment in one of the most secure rental apartment complexes in Fort Lauderdale. This was a big transition, but it was something she deeply wanted. As I came to learn from Pati, things go much better when the Aspie is involved in the decision-making. Rebecca told us she had found an independent living facility that was farther away but still relatively nearby. A few months later she moved to this campus that provided her with her own apartment, some life coaching, and transportation for those who could not drive.

After moving into her apartment at the facility, she began shopping at the nearby Publix but would go only if her coach accompanied her. Just as Rebecca began to get into a comfort zone for shopping there, her guide-coach had to take a short leave from the independent living facility. Her mentor, Pati, filled in for the coach to take Rebecca shopping, but this change in routine took Rebecca out of her comfort zone. When her coach returned, she drew Rebecca a diagram to serve as a road map of the Publix, which was a big shot in the arm for Rebecca. Not only did she get back into her comfort zone, but she began to feel truly confident in shopping. With this visual Aspertool, she's become more independent with her shopping. Soon she may not think twice about shopping, with or without her coach.

Action Plan: Give your Aspie advance notice and help her prepare if there's going to be a change in the routine or if she will be put into a new environment. Routine is important to her. Think long and hard before you change it. Even when she is in a positive routine, keep your eyes open for any negative habits you might observe your Aspie falling back into; this might be a sign she is slipping out of the routine. And once she falls out of the routine, it can be tough for her to get back into it. But with help, she can do it.

---

16 I once saw on a TV documentary that Costco eschews signage because they know the customer ends up buying some 20 percent more stuff that way.

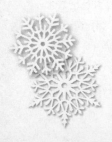

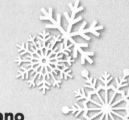

Tip from ESE Teacher Pati Fizzano

A good routine helps Aspies manage their anxiety; it's their survival technique. If Aspies go off their routines, there's a good chance they'll have a meltdown. In school, Aspies have to deal with many types of changes to their routines—half days, classroom changes, standardized testing days. One of the toughest is when their teachers are out sick and there's a substitute. Yikes! Letting them know of such changes a day ahead can make for a smoother transition, but, even then, the changes are still difficult for some Aspies to process.

The number of activities in their routines should be within their comfort levels. For instance, some Aspies may not be able to handle more than three activities in a day.

The earlier you can get your Aspie into a structured routine, the easier life will be for you and your family. Some Aspies accept flexibility only when it benefits them. For instance, if I'm supposed to pick up Rebecca at 12:30 but I am running late, I will call her at noon to say I can't get there until 1:00. Of course, she's fine with that—that means she can stay in her apartment thirty minutes longer. But if I were to call at noon and ask her to be ready five minutes earlier, she would get frustrated and probably have a slight meltdown.

Thought from Rebecca Reitman

I do not place other people's schedules on my calendar. My calendar is only for my stuff, such as doctor appointments, tutoring, and so on. If there's going to be a change to my schedule, such as my coach being away for a few days, I like to know that at least a week in advance, preferably two. If my father is going out of town, it helps if he tells me two weeks prior. Finding out about a change at the last second is a freak-out, but knowing of a change too far in advance is useless. It just makes me more anxious. If I'm told of a change months ahead, I'll probably forget.

The more out of my routine I am, the more anxious I get. Surprises add to my anxiety level. I don't like surprise parties or even big non-surprise parties. When my parents used to throw me birthday parties, they'd invite fifty people, which was way too many for me. I should be able to choose what type of birthday party I'm having.

Also, if I'm going to attend a family get-together, it helps to know in advance the seating plan for dinner. That way I can plan for talking to whomever I'll be sitting next to.

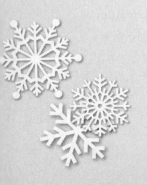

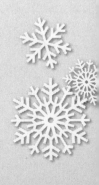

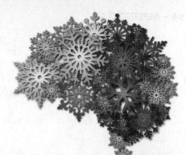

9 STRUCTURE AND POSITIVE ACTIVITIES

> The happiest people are
> those who are too busy to notice
> whether they are or not.
>
> —*William Feather*

Helpful Hint: An Aspie's daily schedule should be marked by structure. Sure, structure is vital for every person, for every type of brain—we all need a full dance card. But it's that much more important for the Aspie. An Aspie who is in a routine that incorporates positive, productive activities is an Aspie who is doing well. Positive activities give Aspies feelings of self-worth and self-esteem, ward off depression, eliminate isolation, and enable them to socialize.

I f things seem to be spiraling out of control for your Aspie, when it seems like there's no clear-cut path for his long-term happiness, the magic bullet is *structure*.

Principle: For Aspies, structure means having a regular place to go and being involved in a productive activity that makes them want to get up in the morning, perform all the morning activities on their checklists, and be on time for the bus. Structure and activities serve to remind Aspies that life is not a one-way street and that there's more to it than just thinking about oneself. It means having a purpose in life. It means being with other people and helping them. Helping others is a part of the ideal structure for an Aspie (as it is for all of us).

A few examples will help illustrate this principle. A friend's son who is an Aspie had been floundering for years. Robbie struggled to finish high school, then started experimenting with marijuana. He ended up in a rehab program. His parents sent him to a series of therapists and other mental health professionals. They even put him in a wilderness program out West. Nothing seemed to work.

Then a friend of the family found Robbie an entry-level job at a hamburger restaurant. He'd get up each morning, shower, shave, put on his work uniform, and drive to his job, where he'd work long hours. It turned out Robbie loved all the structure and the routine activities the job entailed. He'd return home each evening, spend time talking with his folks, watch TV, go to sleep, then get up the next morning and start the routine again.

Now Robbie has straightened out the other aspects of his life: no more drugs, no more drama. On his days off, Robbie goes to movies with friends. At work he's been promoted to assistant manager. He's even thinking of buying his own franchise (with his family's financial assistance). Robbie couldn't be happier, and his folks couldn't be more thrilled.

My daughter, Rebecca, wanted more independence and decided that she didn't like living so close to her parents. She applied to live at a supervised independent living complex about a half-hour drive on the highway away from us.

ESE teacher Pati Fizzano became Rebecca's mentor, coach, and teaching colleague. Rebecca started taking the bus for the disabled to the middle school where she would work alongside Pati each day from 3:30 to 5:45 tutoring, mentoring, and caring for the Aspies in the after-school program. Pati would then drive Rebecca to her house, where Rebecca tutored math in the Individualized Education Program (IEP) for private high school and college students with similar learning challenges, including Asperger's. In these one-on-one sessions, which sometimes go for over three hours per student, Rebecca uses her gifts to reach, teach, and inspire students whose brains work a bit differently. After the sessions, Pati would drive Rebecca back to the independent living facility.

This makes for a long day—for both Pati and Rebecca—with the tutoring sessions often not over until 10:00 PM. But being busy with what she's good at and loves to do gave Rebecca greater self-esteem. Her daily life now had structure, and the more structure there was, the more activities she added. It became a self-fulfilling circle. She got into the flow of life. Of course, the tutoring activities involved socialization as well. So for Rebecca, all the dots started to connect.

After Ralph couldn't make college work out for him, he returned to his parents' home to live. Ralph had tried to go away to college but couldn't go through with it because his friend, who was also supposed to attend, cancelled at the last minute. So Ralph went to a local state school and lived at home. This proved to be a bad situation. Ralph was socially awkward, and he slept in every day. Because he was isolated and not doing anything constructive, he became somewhat depressed. His well-meaning parents watched helplessly as their son with Asperger's stagnated.

Luckily, Ralph's dad called in a favor and got his son a job at a friend's pizzeria as a delivery man. It turned out to be his dream job. It provided just the right amount of socialization and taught Ralph about responsibility and earning money. And the hours suit him to a tee, because he still likes to sleep through until late morning. His parents can now focus on other adolescence- and Aspie-related battles.

Action Plan: Structure and activities go hand in hand. You can't allow your Aspie to become isolated, sitting alone in his room, whether at the computer, watching TV, or listening to music. Being alone in his room on a computer does not count as structure. He must interact with others, help others when possible, and fill up the days with worthwhile activities. Try to harness your Aspie's interests into positive activities, such as a job, a hobby, a sport or recreational activity, volunteering at a nursing home or a youth center, or helping out at school. Structured activities are the foundation for a happy and fulfilling life for all of us, but especially for the unique individuals we call Aspies.

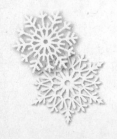

Tip from ESE Teacher Pati Fizzano

Parents and teachers must set expectations and goals for their Aspies. This is nonnegotiable! If parents don't get their Aspies to interact with other people, both inside and outside the home, their Aspies will become only more antisocial and lead a more hermit-like existence.

Start by sitting down with them at an early age and using a visual, such as a calendar, to set up a schedule of fun activities. Change it weekly until you find the right fit. If your Aspie starts getting stubborn about not taking part in the activity, remain firm (but loving). Give it time to sink in. Don't give up. Aspies love consistency, no matter what their ages.

Remember, Aspies are rule followers. Design a structure for their activities, and include rewards to back up their participation and achievements.

Thought from Rebecca Reitman

I don't know if parents should push their Aspies to take part in group activities. But if they choose to do so, they need to be aware of crossing the line and being unreasonable in what they're asking of their Aspies. Putting too much on an Aspie's plate will only create more anxiety.

Your Aspie may not be able to handle the pace you want him to improve at when taking part in activities. Keep in mind that your Aspie may be making steady improvements, but it's possible that these improvements are too subtle, slow, or gradual for you to notice.

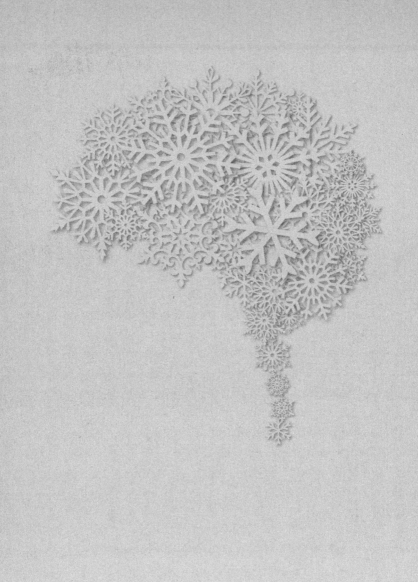

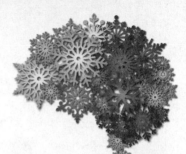

10 OBSESSIONS AND HYPER-INTERESTS

> Passion is energy.
> Feel the power that comes
> from focusing on what
> excites you.
>
> —*Oprah Winfrey*

Helpful Hint: The way Aspies' brains are hardwired, they are going to find one or two (or maybe more) areas that really interest them and focus on those areas intensely. Some people call these obsessions; I call them hyper-interests. If the hyper-interest is a positive one, it should be harnessed and encouraged.

Growing up with Charlie in the Greenville section of Jersey City, I got to know him at an early age. Our fathers played gin together twice a week. Charlie and I would pal around, mostly at the Jewish Community Center, where we'd play basketball for hours on end.

Charlie was quiet, serious, cerebral, and kept to himself. I was a boisterous, backslapping, classic Type A personality and had the much larger social circle. But despite our different personalities, we became close friends at Snyder High School and even formed our own little Sherlock Holmes group, which we called the Diogenes Club. We discussed cases, used our powers of observation, and tried to create and figure out little mysteries for ourselves.

Looking back at those years from my current perspective, I can now see a bit of Aspieness in Charlie. Maybe it was that he was a private person who never wasted words. Maybe it was his genius IQ. Maybe it was his love of numbers. But when I say he loved numbers, I'm not talking about discrete math. The numbers Charlie loved to study were the ones in the racing forms. You see, Charlie was obsessed with the trotters—the sport of harness racing. Maybe he'd gotten the bug from his father, who worked at Yonkers Raceway but always tried to dissuade his son from going into that area. I also tried to convince Charlie that gambling was a waste of time, especially for someone as smart as he was. But the trotters were his obsession, his hyper-interest.

Charlie and I were teammates on Snyder's varsity basketball team. Charlie's court savvy and awareness made him one of the top guards in Hudson County. After graduation, we both went to college in Boston—me to Boston University for its six-year medical program (despite having been expelled from school twice along the way, making me wonder how I would have been labeled growing up), Charlie to Brandeis on an academic scholarship. That winter our schools' basketball teams played each other. Charlie was captain of the Brandeis freshman team (then coached by legendary Boston Celtic K.C. Jones), while I came off the bench for BU.

After the game, Charlie and I got together and talked about our plans. I asked Charlie if he was still obsessed with going to the track and betting on the horses. "Of course, Hack," he said. "What did you expect?"

"Charlie, when are you going to give this up? You have the highest IQ of anyone I know. There must be a thousand things a smart guy like you could do. And you're never going to get the chance, because you're going to flunk out of college." I figured that all the time he was spending at the track had to be affecting his grades—though it did not. I continued, "Face it. You're never going to make a living at the track."

He didn't argue; he was never one to waste words. He just smiled.

Well, as I've said throughout this book, I was once clueless about Asperger's and I was just as clueless when giving Charlie career advice. Charlie Singer harnessed (no pun intended) his obsession and went on to become a top handicapper of the trotters at the Meadowlands Racetrack in East Rutherford, New Jersey. For years he set the morning lines there. His peers respected him for his handicapping skills,[17] and his coworkers loved him. One of them said that Charlie was the only guy he knew who "could watch a race once with binoculars and see everything."

In August 1989 Charlie was diagnosed with non-Hodgkin's lymphoma. He worked on and off until he succumbed to the cancer four years later. Just four months after his premature death at age fifty-three, the first Charles Singer Memorial harness race was run at Meadowlands.

Principle: There's a fine line between interests and obsessions. Your Aspie may become obsessed with a certain activity or an area. She'll eat, live, and sleep it—as well as talk about it nonstop. She will want to tell everyone about it but won't have the patience to listen to others talk about their interests. She'll go on and on until the person she's talking to walks away. (Using role-playing, you can help teach them not to be a conversation hog.)

Don't be too quick to dig in your heels and forbid that activity. First, decide if the interest is a positive or negative one. If you can harness the obsession and convert it into a positive interest that can spur the Aspie's productivity and enable her to earn a living, it's a win-win situation. Many Aspies go on to become professionals in the area they obsess on. Silicon Valley companies such as Apple, Google, and SAP have hired and nurtured Aspies, placing great value on their analytical skills and their ability to focus.

Jason had Asperger's syndrome. The educational system in the area where he lived and attended public school was not doing a good job of teaching him. So his mother founded a school that specialized in education for kids with Asperger's syndrome. Jason became one of the first students.

Jason had always been fascinated by cars, particularly General Motors cars. When he was thirteen, he won a Special Olympics event and was given a Toyota baseball cap as a prize. He said he would keep the cap out of respect, but he wanted to go on record to say, "Toyota should come out and recognize once and for all that GM is the real king of the road."

When fifteen-year-old Jason was failing math, Rebecca began tutoring him. She harnessed his obsession with automobiles by teaching his math lessons in terms of cars and car design.

Under Rebecca's tutelage, Jason started doing better at school. But his obsession with cars didn't wane one bit. Most people viewed Jason's car obsession as a problem and tried to shift him to other interests. But a local car dealer who was also a benefactor of Jason's school saw the opportunity to harness Jason's obsession as a win-win situation by giving him a job at his Chevy dealership.

The young Aspie learned to modify his behavior, toned down his rhetoric, and took sales training courses. He read everything he could about selling cars and in particular Chevrolets. In addition, he simply would not let a potential buyer walk off the lot without buying a vehicle; therefore, you'll understand how, in just his third month on the job, fifteen-year-old Jason broke the dealership's sales record by selling thirty-eight vehicles!

Everyone (and particularly Aspies) should be encouraged to discover their passion and then pursue it. If you can make a living at it, and if you can help others while you do it, so much the better. A great woman once said to her son, who she thought was coasting instead of applying himself, "You have a moral obligation to work to your full potential with the gifts that God has given you, to help yourself, your family, your friends, and those less fortunate. And to have a good time doing it." That woman was my mother, Evelyn. The son she didn't think was living up to his potential was me. And I've never forgotten the lesson she imparted.

Action Plan: When you're helping your Aspie choose activities, no matter what her age, don't dig in your heels and make her exclude the area she's obsessed with. Try to harness that hyper-interest, turn it into a positive, and give her a chance to live her dreams.

---

17 If Charlie said something and you didn't get it, that was your problem. He wouldn't waste time explaining it. Once he was on vacation in Florida and took me to the track with him. He said, "Hack, I'm on vacation, I'm just out to have a good time. Don't ask me who I like." I agreed, but since he was Charlie Singer, handicapper par excellence, I peeked over his shoulder and saw that in the first race he'd circled the seven horse. I went to the window and put $10 on the seven to win. The horse came in last. In the second race I "noticed" he'd picked the seven horse again. I bet it again. This one finished fifth. In the next two races, Charlie picked the seven. Both lost. Finally I said, "Charlie, why are you picking the seven horse in each race?

He said, "The Mick." Of course! That was the other thing he and I had in common: we both worshipped Mickey Mantle, the immortal number 7 of the New York Yankees.

Charlie had warned me not to ask him which horse he liked. But I didn't listen. He wasn't handicapping that day, he was just having fun. What does this have to do with Aspies? Maybe nothing. Or maybe we should do a little more listening to them and try to understand the way their brains work, rather than impose our will on them.

Tip from ESE Teacher Pati Fizzano

An Aspie's positive obsessions should be harnessed and encouraged. If a child has a positive hyper-interest, the teacher or parents should have the Aspie focus her energy there. You never know where it will lead.

Many of the significant advances in the various sciences and the arts have been made by people who had Asperger's. (It's a fact that many Aspies have the ability to focus for longer periods of time than non-Aspies.) A list of famous people with Asperger's or similar traits would include scientists and inventors Albert Einstein, Thomas Edison, Sir Isaac Newton, Charles Darwin, Alexander Graham Bell, and Benjamin Franklin; Microsoft founder Bill Gates; and business tycoon Howard Hughes. The computer scientist cryptographer who broke the Nazi secret Enigma code in World War II, Alan Turing, has recently been depicted in the award-winning movie *The Imitation Game*.

In the arts the names would include the artists Vincent van Gogh and Michelangelo; composers Beethoven and Mozart; authors Mark Twain and George Orwell; director Alfred Hitchcock; actors Robin Williams and Dan Aykroyd; puppeteer Jim Henson; and cartoonist Charles Schulz.

Other famous people include U.S. presidents Thomas Jefferson and Abraham Lincoln; animal behaviorist Temple Grandin, who is a speaker and author about the topic of autism; and Hans Asperger, the pediatrician and medical theorist after whom Asperger's syndrome is named.

However, not all obsessions are positive. What the Aspie is focusing on or obsessing about can be negative, such as watching violent movies or playing violent video games. Even playing nonviolent video games can become a negative obsession, because they can become addictive. Nearly all of my Aspie students are obsessed with playing games on their phones or computers. They admit that they play these games through the night, sometimes until early morning.

Aspies like playing video games for many reasons. First of all, it can be a social pastime for them. If they play online they can meet "friends," and these people accept them for who they are. Aspies generally have a hard time meeting and keeping friends. They don't understand how to enter or exit a conversation, and they feel awkward around people. When they're playing video games online, Aspies don't have to worry about their lack of social skills.

In addition, when they play video games they feel like they're "in control." They set goals (i.e., moving to higher levels in the game) and try to achieve them. They also like the repetition of the video game. Finally, after being in school or a work setting all day, video games allow them to stay in their safe place and be comfortable.

Many parents encourage their Aspies to play games on their computers so that they can get a break. For example, the mother of a six-year-old I'd worked with came to me to discuss her son. He had already been kicked out of several schools because of his behavior issues. She admitted that she often "rewarded" her son by letting him play video games in his room for as much as two hours a night; she felt this was her only time for getting her things done.

I said to her, "If he's getting two hours of game time a night at age six, how much will he be getting when he's twelve?"

I try to limit computer time as much as possible, because I know how addictive computer games are. In fact, I advise refraining from using unmonitored computer time as a reward. I like to reward my students with a team-building lesson, where they play board games with friends. Since most board games involve at least two players, they learn to take turns and play by the rules. It's a reward that helps them learn about fairness.

Thought from Rebecca Reitman

As Aspie's positive interests should definitely be harnessed and encouraged. When I was a child, I was a distance runner and was able to successfully harness that drive and determination to make the all-county team as a high school cross-country athlete. I also spent countless hours working math problems and subsequently was a math tutor to other students. I went on to major in math at college and work today tutoring math to children up to college-aged students.

I have a different outlook on computer activities. I don't think video games are necessarily negative. Better to be playing them than doing drugs or engaging in criminal acts. When Aspies are on their computers, they're rebooting . . . and getting some needed alone time.

As far as guidelines about content or time, judge your child on an individual basis to determine this. If your child is hard-working, then she probably understands the ramifications of not getting her work done and needs no limits or guidelines. On the other hand, you might have a student who is a genius but also lazy and will do things her way no matter what you say. Perhaps a third party, such as a psychologist, could help decide what is appropriate. Again, every brain is different, and your powers of observation are your best place to start.

It's fine to introduce Aspies to potential new interests. But don't take away their one true hyper-interest. That's their security blanket.

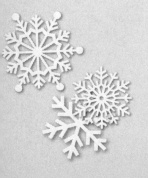

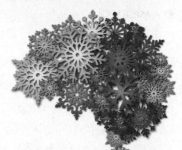

11 SOCIAL AWKWARDNESS

> Friendship is the only thing
> in the world concerning the usefulness
> of which all mankind is agreed.
>
> — *Cicero*

Helpful Hint: As they go through life, Aspies need the same social skills as any other member of society. But because of their social awkwardness, they have a hard time developing these skills. It's your job to make sure they get the training that will enable them to socialize to the best of their abilities. Preparation, role-playing, and practice are important tools to help them learn socialization skills.

Principle: Call it a stereotype or defining trait, but if there's one constant among individuals with Asperger's syndrome, it's that they have a hard time socializing. They're socially awkward and uncomfortable around people. Many of them prefer being alone, in their rooms, often at their computers. (Remember, one size doesn't fit all. Some folks with Aspie traits do just fine socially. If your Aspie is doing well in social situations, that's great. Remember what I said about who am I calling an Aspie. If a chapter or an Aspertool works, use it. If not, just skip it.)

When they're young children, most Aspies want lots of friends. But they soon learn it's hard to make friends and hard to keep them if they don't know how to start a conversation (or end one). Playdates with non-Aspies can be tense affairs; the Aspie tends to follow rules, and if the playmate doesn't, the Aspie may get frustrated and start a fight. Even a playdate with two Aspies can be a challenge; some parents of Aspies don't like to have other Aspies over because of the potential meltdowns. (Of course, these parents may not want to admit to themselves, let alone others, that their children have any label, let alone Asperger's. One reason for this book is to tackle the unintentional cluelessness that's out there at every level, from society at large to the parents of Aspies themselves. I include myself as a former totally clueless parent who is now just a little bit less clueless.)

If an Aspie's repeated attempts at socializing result in a series of psychological smackdowns, he will understandably retreat to the comfort zone of solitude. Give Aspies the choice of engaging in an activity that forces them to leave that womb, and they'll in all likelihood refuse.

So your goal is to provide safe situations in which Aspies can practice social skills and even socialize to some degree. You'll have to provide these situations gradually. The more organized activities you can get Aspies into at an early age, the better their social development will be. A dance class is doubly beneficial, because it helps with their physicality and coordination and brings them together with other kids. Organized sports that are safe (I don't condone dangerous sports like boxing, motor racing, or football) and properly coached are also a possibility for many Aspies. Rebecca was a cross-country runner and also played softball. Any sport with a deep regimen can help them succeed, because they typically like the repetitiveness. Controlled sleepovers can be beneficial.

(To this day, my adult daughter rarely misses an opportunity to remind me that when she was a child, her mom and I did not allow her to experience social situations, such as sleepovers, on her own often enough. She cuts us no slack over our concern back then over the twenty-three vascular tumors in her brain, her two life-saving [against all odds] brain surgeries, her seizure disorder, her extremely trusting and naïve nature, and the meanness of some other kids. When I protest, she quickly adds, "Dad, if you don't want the truth, don't ask.")

When Aspies start going to school, their teachers will hopefully instruct them in socialization skills. Mainstreaming refers to the practice of educating students with special needs in regular classes during specific time periods based on their skill levels. School is a mainstreaming activity for the Aspie, but it can be a challenging environment. Teachers, even those in the special needs area, are often not as knowledgeable as they could be about the specifics of Asperger's. Many classmates can be cruel and will pick on another kid who is socially inept. Bottom line: many problems are associated with the admirable practice of mainstreaming.

On the other hand, some Aspie students are able to initiate interactions with other students. They may exhibit the need to take control and direct social situations according to their own social rules and limited social understanding. This means that these interactions do not constitute a true give-and-take social relationship; they primarily relate to the Aspie's wants, needs, and interests. One of the harder lessons many Aspies need to learn is that "it's not all about you." (This is a criticism that applies to many of us—people direct it at me all the time. It just shows that, as with all the behaviors discussed in this book, they apply to all of us to some degree, but they are amplified in the Aspie.)

Action Plan: Aspies need to be taught appropriate social skills and interactions. They need to be shown how their words and actions impact others. Parents and teachers must realize that the Aspie may not understand common social interactions, may not get jokes, and may be unable to interpret body language. They may have to teach Aspies what social cues mean in order to help them make friends. They may try to improve an Aspie's understanding of social interactions and emotional relationships through visual Aspertools, such as "social stories" and "social scripts," as well as conversations depicted in comic strip format. One of the best Aspertools for this is role-playing—practicing social situations.

Since many Aspies prefer not to socialize, it's your responsibility to get them with other people. Mainstream them where possible, but, at the very least, get them into safe situations with other nice people. Will they make friends? Find romance? Get married one day? These are all possibilities, but not if they're sitting in their rooms by themselves. "You can't hit a home run unless you step up to the plate and swing the bat," is how Paul Kaliades, my lifelong friend and fellow Jersey City stickball player, put it. Of course, if your Aspie doesn't want to step up to the plate, it's your responsibility to nudge him there.

Imagine you're an Aspie. You are twenty-three and your parents have talked you into going to a party, saying you'll have a good time. As you walk into a room full of strangers, your hyper-senses are assaulted by a rush of noises and smells. So many conversations at once, and everyone is wearing a pungent cologne or perfume. The lights are flashing. Your brain is being pummeled on many fronts, and the effect on your nerves is like someone running his fingernails down a blackboard.

A couple invades your personal space and begins asking you questions, making jokes, gesturing. You can't read their verbal cues or their body language. When you try to take part in the conversation, you take everything they say literally. You're way off base. You start talking about your interests and you don't know when to stop because you can't read their cues. Finally the couple walks away. A distant relative you've met once or twice recognizes you and gives you a big bear hug, then moves on when you do not know how to respond. Your anxiety is going through the roof. But no one can tell, because they're not looking at your repetitive hand movements. They don't notice your smile is phony. You're exhausted and humiliated. You can't cope with this right now. Why can't your folks understand that it's easier for you to sit alone in your room?

Socialization is possible for Aspies. Henry was an Aspie who, after graduating high school, stayed home alone every day for six months straight. He had no desire to socialize with anyone. Finally his worried parents learned of a nearby meet-up group for Aspies. It took them several weeks of coaxing, but they finally convinced their son to go. Henry met some peers and discovered he actually liked the experience of socializing. Now he goes to the group weekly and meets with other Aspies. His socialization skills are improving, and he's developing friendships.

A friend's twenty-one-year-old son, Joel, had fully retreated into his comfort zone of solitude. To pry his son out of his room, the father got Joel a job at a small family-owned restaurant. Joel enjoyed his work and began to blossom. He made friends with some of the other employees. He liked earning money. It was a turning point in his life. He is now much more comfortable socially, is pursuing other activities, and wants to move up the ladder at work.

Action Plan: Getting your Aspie to take part in a safe activity with nice people is infinitely preferable to his sitting alone in his room. In fact, learning socially acceptable behavior so he can have positive interactions with other individuals is mandatory. Training and role-playing are key Aspertools for getting your Aspie to socialize. Start small, with Asperger's meet-up groups, which provide structure and daily activities for participants. Then consider moving up to groups of people with similar interests, like a book club, a movie club, or even a writer's club. Getting a job can be a real game changer—it's the equivalent of throwing him into the socialization pool headfirst. But the bottom line is that whatever gets him into the presence of other people in a nurturing and productive manner is a plus.

Never give up. An Aspie's social skills can be improved at any age, even well into adulthood. Adult Aspies also have plenty of potential to grow into change. Let's not discriminate against Aspies because of their calendar age.

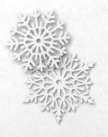

Tip from ESE teacher Pati Fizzano

It is important for the Aspie to learn social skills. Our curriculum teaches children with autism step-by-step lessons in social awareness. Each lesson plan is told through social stories, role-playing, and group activities.

We begin the school year by showing students a visual that I designed called The Six Steps of Friendship Ladder.

Step 1: The Hello Stage

When you meet someone for the first time. You introduce yourself, but don't give too much personal information, which might scare a new friend away.

Step 2: The Exchanging Stage

You become a little friendlier and exchange phone numbers, e-mail addresses, etc.

Step 3: The Meeting Stage

You're becoming closer friends. You might meet at the movies or go out to lunch together.

Step 4: The Playing Stage

You invite your friend over to your house. (Parents may want to supervise this playdate and set a time limit to the playdate. Too much togetherness may be too much for the Aspie to handle.)

Step 5: The Trusting Stage

You begin to trust your friend with secrets.

Step 6: The Best Friend Stage

You consider this friend your best friend. You'll be there to support him and help if he needs you.

I explain all six stages and tell the students that the steps don't happen overnight. A student once came running into my classroom and said, "Ms. Fizz, I just made a new best friend!" I took him to the Steps of Friendship wall and asked him to point out which step that was. He pointed to Step 6 and said, "Oops, I missed steps one through five."

Thought from Rebecca Reitman

It's important to set goals for Aspies, especially in terms of their socialization skills. But the biggest mistake parents and teachers make in trying to get an Aspie to socialize is that they don't understand how the Aspie's brain works. Parents and teachers will treat an Aspie like a non-Aspie. This is why many parents become frustrated. Remember, I wasn't diagnosed with Asperger's until three years past my college graduation. My dad, for instance, didn't realize why I wouldn't do certain things and yelled at me in frustration or got discouraged.

Teachers can also hinder the Aspie's education or progress in socializing by calling him dumb or giving him a wrong label. Some schools give up on Aspies by not letting them think outside the box.

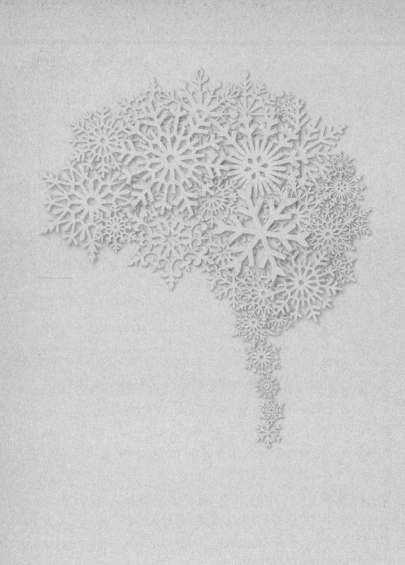

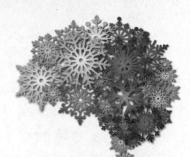

12 LIMIT CHOICES TO AVOID "NO!"

> When you make a choice,
> you change the future.
>
> — *Deepak Chopra*

Helpful Hint: If you ask your Aspie if she wants to try a new activity or interact with someone new, her answer will always be no. She is comfortable in her known routine. Asking her open-ended questions with an infinite number of possible answers won't work either—that will just overwhelm her. For the best result, restate the question in a way that limits her choices.

Principle: The thought of doing anything different, or anything that involves interacting with other people, causes Aspies anxiety. Ask your Aspie if she wants to go to a family dinner on Sunday and she'll say, "No." (Maybe "No thanks" if you're lucky.) In fact, if you ask if she wants to do anything outside of her routine, chances are she'll simply respond, "No." Given a choice, she'll always say no.

I t's a tug-of-war. You want your Aspie to expand her comfort zone; she prefers to remain in that zone, within herself, where life is easier and more predictable. If Aspies had their druthers, that's where they'd stay forever—living a hermit-like existence in their rooms, with their computers (which many Aspies think of as their best friends). In this comfort zone, there's not much in the way of social development, but there's a lot less stress and less anxiety.

After Rebecca finished her one-year internship tutoring math at the school for kids with Asperger's, I asked the headmistress what she felt would be the best thing for me to do to help Rebecca going forward. She thought it over, then said, "Hackie, don't give her the choice to say no."

Action Plan: Go back to that question about the family dinner. The Aspertool is to pose that question not as a close-ended yes or no question but as a *multiple-choice question*. I don't mean the type of multiple choice question you often see on an exam, where you can select A, B, C, D, None of the above, or All of the above. I mean something like: "We're going as a family to have dinner with Grandma and Grandpa. Would you rather go Saturday or Sunday?" This makes it easier for Aspies on several counts. First, they don't have to figure out anything. You've already laid down the law— they *are* going to the gathering—so there's no need for discussion of that. All they need to do is pick which day is better. You've made their lives—and yours—less complicated by playing to their preference for specifics.[18]

---

18 This is not to say that multiple choice options always work. I'll never forget the time my mother, Ev, presented my cousin Peter, who was then eleven and maybe sixty pounds soaking wet, with one of her own "multiple choice" options. She was preparing a meal of linguini with white clam sauce for me and three of my Jersey City pals, who would devour anything and everything put in front of them. My cousin, who was your classic picky eater—at this point in his life, he had never even tried tuna fish—took one look at what Ev had made, grimaced, and said he wasn't hungry. If this was his home, his mother would have cooked him a hamburger. But this was not how it worked in my family. Ev told Peter to sit down and eat. Peter said he'd have a bologna sandwich later. Ev said, "Peter, you have two dinner options. You can eat it or you can wear it." Peter took another look at the pasta swimming in canned clam sauce and said, "Aunt Evelyn, I really can't eat that." My mother grabbed his bowl and dumped the contents on his head.

Tip from ESE Teacher Pati Fizzano

Making decisions less complicated for Aspies is the right idea, but you also want to train them to make choices on their own. Many Aspies get overwhelmed by the menu at a restaurant. One cure for this is to talk about the menu before you go to the restaurant or pull it up online and let them view it in advance. This will eliminate the anxiety that might occur at the restaurant.

One of my students asked for an easy way of picking out a movie to see with his family. I told him to take the movie section from the paper and cut out all the names of the ones he'd be allowed to see, put all the titles in a hat, and pull out two of them. Then choose one of those two "finalists." He said, "That's a pretty cool way of doing it."

Aspies struggle with making choices. Teachers of Aspies need to help them learn strategies for getting through life. Easier decision-making is part of that. Remember that most Aspies are shy, and when they are asked a question, the easiest thing for them to do is to say no. So rather than asking a yes-or-no question like "Do you want to go to the movies with Daddy and me?" give them specific choices by asking, "Would you rather see Movie A or Movie B?"

Thought from Rebecca Reitman

As a parent, you must help your Aspie make decisions, particularly when it comes to socializing, but you must also realize when it is in your (and your Aspie's) best interest to step back a bit. Give her choices—real choices, not just what you may have fabricated to fit your agenda—but not too many, just a few at a time. Even if you're well-intentioned, you may think that you are right and she is wrong. You may also expect an Aspie to improve socially at a much faster pace than is possible.

At times Aspies may need a different member of her team to help her out. And sometimes, when another member of the team does get involved, you may not realize just how far your child has gotten, thanks to that other person. I used to be a hermit, but now I socialize with the people I live with, lead and attend activities, and have a job helping others. My family at the place where I live understands the huge progress I have made, even when that progress was just incremental steps, and sometimes more than my biological family understands. The Aspertools of patience and understanding are just two of the essential skills you must develop. You may have to repeat socialization lessons many times over, but know that your Aspie is trying, even if the progress is not apparent to you.

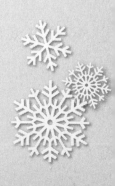

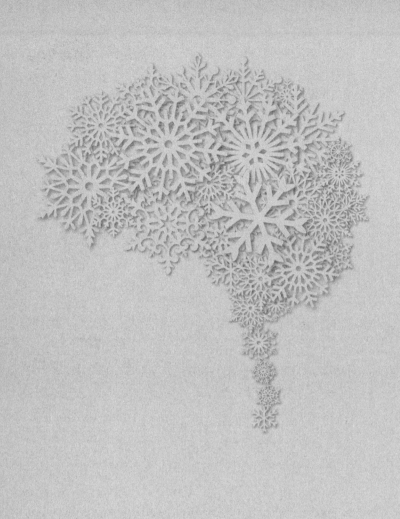

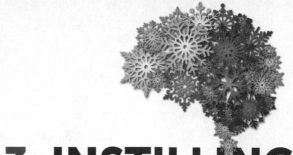

13 INSTILLING STREET SMARTS

> Being street smart comes from experience. It means you've learned how to take what has happened to you, good or bad, and learn to improve from it.
>
> —*Scott Berkun*

Helpful Hint: The ways of the world don't come naturally to Aspies. They lack street smarts and most survival instincts. They can't tell the good guys from the bad guys. They can be quite gullible and easily swayed (except, of course, by their parents). To protect themselves, they'll need to be taught the logic of day-to-day situations in a way their brain circuitry can process. Teaching and insisting on ironclad rules will be helpful, because then they won't have any decisions to make. Providing a safe mechanism for gaining experience is also a key tactic.

Principle: Aspies lack the neurotypical's instincts for self-preservation and survival, as well as their other common-sense tendencies. But they must be trained to survive in the world as it is. Your job is to teach them the logic (or at least the mechanics) of the actions that don't come naturally to them, particularly street smarts.

Sure, it's generalizing to say that all Aspies are gullible. After all, Aspies' brains are all different, and your Aspie may have a healthy dose of common sense. But many don't. If the shoe fits, wear it. On "the street," the downside of making a mistake is huge.

Following is a tragic example of what can happen on the streets. Andrew Young, a forty-year-old man with Asperger's syndrome, spoke several languages, but, according to his family, he had the social skills of a fourteen-year-old. Andrew's friends described him as someone who "wouldn't hurt a fly."

On November 6, 2013, Andrew was walking on the sidewalk in Bournemouth, England, when a bicyclist rode very close to him. He told the bicyclist that riding on the sidewalk was dangerous. It's not that what he said was incorrect, but, because he lacked social skills, the comment came off as sounding arrogant and rude, which apparently didn't sit well with the cyclist and his friends. The cyclist rode away, but a cohort walking behind him sucker-punched the Aspie flush in the face. Young collapsed and hit his head on the pavement. He died the following day at a hospital from his head injury, his mother at his side. The man who threw the punch on the gentle Aspie pleaded guilty to manslaughter and received a prison term of four and a half years.

This demonstrates the importance of giving the Aspie ironclad rules. If they have a rule to fall back on, they don't have to figure out each specific situation. (Keep in mind that teaching Aspies can be frustrating; they'll want to focus on the specific example, while you're interested in establishing a general, easy-to-follow rule they can apply to many situations.) Rules reduce the Aspie's daily anxiety level. Once a rule is set in stone, it gives the Aspie a trusted Aspertool to rely on when a situation arises.

One rule might be that if you're out in public and you need help, go to someone wearing a uniform or someone at their job— for example, a store employee at the mall. Aspies must be told, "Never go to a stranger for help!" Similarly, if a stranger comes up to them and asks for help, they should walk away. Strangers do not approach children for assistance. As with many things, the lines get blurred as your Aspie journeys toward adulthood.

But the street smart rules you try to hand down to your Aspie don't apply to what to do just when he's outside. Plenty of bad things can happen to anyone inside their homes.

Imagine you're an Aspie. The phone rings and you answer it. The man with a gentle voice on the other end identifies himself as Sgt. Smith of the local police department and says that you have to give him your Social Security number for their files. Had you not been trained, you'd have gladly given this nice-sounding man your Social Security number. After all, he's a policeman, a recognized authority figure, and he sounds kind.

But you have been trained! You know the rule is that you are *never ever* to give out your SSN or any confidential information over the phone or on the Internet without checking with a trusted, caring person, such as a parent or your coach. If asked for such information, you simply say, "Not at this time. I have to check with my mom," then call someone you trust and ask for advice. If you follow this rule, you can't be verbally bullied or manipulated. You'll be safe. The rule makes a call like this a non-issue instead of an anxiety-laden stressful situation. You didn't even have to factor in if the caller was a friend or the phone company or a collection agency.

The Internet provides challenges for many of us. Its many phishing scams try to trick you into clicking on a fraudulent link, resulting in malware viruses, or malicious e-mails hope to fool you into giving up your confidential information. One simple rule (and this applies to every Internet user) is never to click on such a link, always to go to the main website of the alleged company that sent you such an e-mail, or to have somebody to go for advice. It is easier to have a rule than to have to figure out each particular situation.

Another rule might be that your Aspie is not allowed to use a credit card on the Internet. The problem with setting this rule is that many Aspies prefer shopping online because it's less stressful than getting to a store and then dealing with a clerk and buying the merchandise there. But it's an easy-to-follow blanket rule that could save a lot of grief. One option you might offer your Aspie is to use prepaid gift cards online. Or maybe the rule might start out as no unsupervised time on the Internet and then evolve into something more flexible. (The Internet poses unique problems for Aspies. For instance, many think they can make friends on the Internet, and if for some reason they need to "tune them off," they can easily do so. But that's not always the case.)

Action Plan: Don't put your Aspie in a bubble. Teach him everything he needs to know. Don't hide anything from him. But create clear and specific rules to protect your Aspie in certain situations, and then strictly enforce those rules. Safety while gaining experience is the goal.

Make sure your Aspie has someone besides you to go to for advice—a trusted individual or group. Teach him the basic "why" of the actions he is to take, using logic that his brain circuitry can follow. This will substitute for his missing instincts. You can even try to teach him street smarts, but keep in mind you'll have to deal with your Aspie's unique brain circuitry.

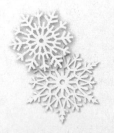

Tip from ESE Teacher Pati Fizzano

Parents need to impress upon their Aspies the importance of money and the ability to count it. Every one of my Aspie students has trouble counting and making change—even those in advanced math. I posed this problem to my students in the Algebra II honors class: "If I gave you a five-dollar bill to purchase a seventy-five-cent candy bar, what change should I get back?" They were giving me back twenties, tens, fives . . . They really struggle with the concept of making change. Carrying cash around is an ongoing problem for them.

There are many possible reasons for this. One, they may never had the exposure to money because their parents may not have given them the opportunity to use it. Another reason is that dealing with money puts them on the spot. Or maybe they never learned how to count up. If they were asked to solve a math problem on paper involving making change, they could do it. But when they have to handle money—when it's physically in their hands, all these different kinds of money, the pennies, nickels, dimes, quarters, dollar bills, five-dollar bills—it's too much information for them and too much pressure, especially if someone is standing over them.

Aspies need to be taught right from wrong like every other child. However, Aspies may need to have it explained a little clearer. Employ the principle of clarity, specificity, and accountability.

Clarity means communicate exactly what you mean; don't walk on eggshells or beat around the bush. Specificity means putting exact numbers to everything: the exact time, the exact date, the exact budget. Accountability means that you cannot have rewards or consequences unless there is specific accountability. I try to ingrain this mantra in everyone, but it especially applies to Aspies.

Street smarts should be taught to all children, especially those on the spectrum. In our socialization class, we role-play with our students to teach them aspects of street smarts. The lesson on Internet dangers takes more than a week. We know that Aspies love computers and feel safe on them. The friends they can't make in the real world they often can find on the computer. I now ask my students what they would do in the following scenario:

You meet someone online—Sally—and learn that both of you share many common interests. Sally asks your age, and you say you're thirteen. What a coincidence! Sally is also thirteen. She asks which school you attend and what grade you're in. You're both in eighth grade, and in another coincidence, Sally lives in the same town as you, but attends the school on the other side of town. The dialogue continues for weeks. You think you've finally grasped the steps of making friends, and now you're building a true friendship. Next, you and Sally exchange pictures, so now you know what Sally looks like—a typical thirteen-year-old girl. Now she suggests the two of you meet next Saturday for lunch at a place within walking distance of your house. You say yes. Why not? Sally's your new BFF. She asks what you'll be wearing and you tell her; then you ask her what she'll be wearing. Turns out the two of you even dress alike.

The day comes and you're excited finally to be meeting Sally. When you get to the meeting spot, an older man comes up to you, smiles, and says, "Hi. You must be Wendy, I'm Sally's father. Sally's running late today and asked me to come pick you up so you don't have to wait for her."

I asked my students, "In this situation, would you get into the car?" Every one of them said yes, because the man knew their name and his daughter was their friend. I finished the story by role-playing the situation with the man abducting the child.

Parents should monitor their children on the computer all the time. They should not let their children have computers in their bedrooms. An article I once read really opened my eyes. It asked parents if they would let a stranger walk into their child's bedroom. No? Then don't leave a computer in your child's bedroom.

Thought from Rebecca Reitman

Don't hide anything from your Aspie just because he's an Aspie. But when explaining things to him, use logic that works with his Aspie brain or for his particular situation. For instance, don't use an example about driving a car if he can't drive, because it will make no sense to him. If the Aspie does not see the logic, he will look for a way around it, or he might try to trick you. I suggest pairing the logic with the things or people that interest him—his "obsessions."

The time to start teaching your Aspie children street smarts is when they're young, because that's when they're still listening to you.

One tip related to shopping: Aspies prefer having gift cards rather than credit cards. A gift card frees us from having to carry around a lot of cash. And if we're using the gift card to shop online, we can buy things without having to divulge our personal banking information.

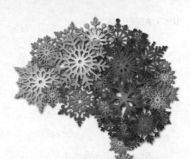

14 TAKING THINGS LITERALLY: "WHY DID THEY SAY I'M NOT PLAYING WITH A FULL DECK?"

One morning I shot an elephant
in my pajamas. How he got into my
pajamas I'll never know.

—*Groucho Marx as Captain Spaulding in*
Animal Crackers.

Helpful Hint: Aspies take everything literally that is said to them or that they read. Not only that, they can't figure out when they're not supposed to take things literally. Be judicious in your choice of idioms and colloquialisms. When you use one, teach the Aspie what it means. Teach them as they occur.

Principle: Many Aspies interpret the words said to them (and, perhaps to a lesser extent, the words they read) quite literally. Consider all the things you might say in jest or exaggeration during the course of a day. *I'm bending over backward to please you. That trip to the supermarket cost me an arm and a leg. They're dropping like flies. He was so wound up, he was bouncing off the walls. I've got an axe to grind with him.* Who'd believe that anyone could take them literally?

Well, don't let their high IQs fool you. Aspies could. And will. The idioms, colloquialisms, exaggerations, and folksy figures of speech that account for so much of our spoken language are confusing to Aspies because they take them literally.

Imagine you're an Aspie. You're waiting for a meeting to start. The neurotypicals next to you are joking around. They're trying to include you, but you're not comfortable being around them because you can't tell when they're being serious and when they're not. You're not sure when to laugh. Someone says, "Janet said if her boss gives her one more stupid assignment, she's gonna blow her top!" and starts laughing. Why is everyone laughing? My dad uses the expression "blowing my top" to refer to my having a meltdown. Why is the idea of someone else blowing their top funny?

Imagine you're an Aspie. You're driving your car and you've gotten lost. Even though you're nineteen and know you shouldn't talk to strangers, you pull over and ask a kindly looking older couple for directions to 508 Main Street. The man smiles and says, "You can't get there from here." Awkward pause. Is that supposed to be funny? Are you supposed to ask the question again? Or are you supposed to backtrack all the way to where you started from to get where you're going? The seconds seem like minutes. The person is still smiling. What should you do next?

Imagine you're an Aspie. You are at a party and the guy you're talking to says he's just pulling your leg. But your leg is in your pants and no one's pulling on it. Are you supposed to laugh? Now someone else says, "Hey, look outside, it's raining cats and dogs!" You look out the window for animals falling from the sky, but all you see are sheets of rain. As your anxiety climbs, your brain can't function to figure out things that it could normally figure out.

Action Plan: It would be easier if you said exactly what you meant in the first place, without resorting to a figure of speech. But that won't prepare Aspies for the real world, where people use idioms and colloquialisms all the time. (The same applies to teaching them how to read body language and social cues.) If you or someone else uses an idiomatic expression or a colloquialism in talking to your Aspie, explain the literal translation of the phrase. Teach your Aspie the most common colloquialisms used in the real world, and explain to her what they mean.

"I don't know what I don't know."

Rebecca felt that her apartment in Fort Lauderdale was too close to her well-intentioned parents, whose tyranny she was trying to escape.[19] After she learned of the independent living facility and had researched it on her own, she asked if she could move there.

Her decision took her mom and me by surprise. The clueless parents were about to become a little bit less clueless. Rebecca had figured that for her to maximize her independence, she needed to find a place where she could have her own apartment yet receive some third-party coaching (not from her parents!), help with transportation, since she did not drive, and a resident manager with special training. The facility was on a campus that included an administration building, an auditorium, a few small parochial schools, and other programs.

During the application process, Rebecca e-mailed Kate, the supervisor of the independent living facility, to ask if there was shopping within walking distance of the facility, because her seizure disorder prevented her from driving. Kate e-mailed back that there were so many shopping centers and stores close by that it might be easier for her to list the ones that *weren't* nearby. She then listed fifteen stores she thought Rebecca would like to shop at that were easy to walk to.

Kate had cc'd me on the e-mail, and the next day as I was driving Rebecca, I said, "Wasn't that nice of Kate to list all those stores you could walk to if you lived there?"

"Dad, you really ought to read your e-mails more carefully. The list Kate sent me is of the stores that are *not* close by," Rebecca said.

Without thinking, I replied, "Rebecca, it wouldn't make sense for her to list the stores that are not close by. You must know that."

I watched my daughter's body language instantly change. She slumped in the passenger seat. Her shoulders sagged, and she muttered, "Dad, that's the problem. Sometimes I don't know what I don't know."

My heart sank. In that moment, I truly realized how difficult it must be for my daughter or any other Aspie. *"I don't know what I don't know"* has to be a cause of terrible anxiety. It means that one minute they can be confident that they clearly understand what's going on in a given situation, only to discover the next minute that they're way off base. What a shock that must be. Yet as bad as Rebecca felt, she felt worse when she saw the disappointment and the sadness on the face of her father—the same father who spoke without thinking.

(Reliving this moment always makes me sad. But it also makes me glad that I'm writing this book, so that you, the reader, will gain some of these clues that I wish I'd had back then. Just remember, it's not about you. It's about your Aspie.)

Not knowing what you don't know can be really, really tough. But keep in mind that Aspies *can and do learn*. There is hope. There are Aspertools. Give them the opportunity to learn the tools they need. They can do it. As actress Darby Stanchfield utters in her brilliant portrayal of a college student Aspie in the movie *The Square Root of 2*, "Dad, have a little faith."

When Rebecca was growing up, she often said, "Dad, have confidence in me." It's a double-edged sword for a parent, because we all want to protect our children, but if we coddle them too much, they won't learn from their failures and mistakes. This is magnified when you are the parent of an Aspie. On the one hand, Rebecca would think, "My dad thinks I can do things that my brain can't do." On the other hand, if I tried to coddle and protect her and tell her that I'd understand if she failed, then she'd think, "Dad has no confidence that I can do these things." Again, my advice is to be patient and, as the line in the movie says, have faith!

(When I wrote that line for the screenplay, I cried. I cried again when Darby said it so perfectly on the first take on the set, again when I first heard her say it on the screen, and even now, as I write it for the book.)

---

19 The parents of an Aspie often speak of feeling unwanted by their offspring. While this can certainly be said about the parents of neurotypical teenagers, Aspies can be positively brutal to their parents. Another reason along with speaking their minds in absolute honesty is the anger they feel because their parents don't understand what they're going through.

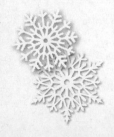

Tip from ESE Teacher Pati Fizzano

Aspies can be taught not to take things literally. At school we use a set of illustrated flash cards, called metaphor cards,[20] to help our Aspies understand the meaning of idioms. One side of the card has the heading "What did you say?" and when you flip the card over it reads, "What did you mean?" Each student keeps a collection of index cards with his or her "personal" idioms. A student might write *It's raining cats and dogs* on one side, then write *It's raining very hard* on the flip side. Once the Aspies feel comfortable with the idiom, we have them use it in conversations, though they're taught that overusing an idiom sounds silly.

Taking things literally has its lighter side too. At the facility where Rebecca lives, maintenance was working on the water pipes. The residence manager told Rebecca to be prepared in case they had to turn off the water. Rebecca went into action. Anything that could hold water she filled up: pots, vases, glasses, measuring cups. When I went to her apartment, I saw vessels filled with water trail from the kitchen through the dining room into the bathroom. After I explained what the residence manager meant, we both had a good laugh.

Thought from Rebecca Reitman

When I hear an idiom I'm not familiar with, I try very hard to figure it out. But most of the time I get it wrong. I wish people would understand my puzzled look and explain the idiom when they use it. The other day my coach said, "You can't teach an old dog new tricks." I assumed she was talking about someone really old learning something new, but I was confused because I knew she was talking about her nineteen-year-old son. I asked why she would say that about someone who's only nineteen. She explained that the idiom doesn't relate to a person's age but is about trying to teach someone something new after they've been doing it their way for a while.

I've found that Aspies who learn idioms when they're younger do better with them later on. Children's brains are like sponges and can absorb so much more than when they get older. When I was a child, the idioms were said to me and explained immediately. I didn't really have a chance to think of the ones introduced to signify something different from their actual meaning.

If an Aspie doesn't know idioms, go over each one until mastery is achieved. Do not be impatient and think the Aspie is not paying attention, as it may take an enormous amount of time for her to understand. Please, do not get discouraged; the Aspie is not faking misunderstanding, for the most part. She really does want to understand.

---

20 Jude Welton *What Did You Say? What Do You Mean? An Illustrated Guide to Understanding Metaphors* (Jessica Kingsley Publishing, 2004).

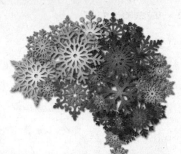

15 SPECIFICS: SAY WHAT YOU MEAN, MEAN WHAT YOU SAY

Words are made for a certain exactness of thought, as tears are made for a certain exactness of pain.

—*Rene D'aumal, French poet*

Helpful Hint: When giving instructions to Aspies, be as specific as possible! Because of the way their brain works, Aspies don't do well with processing vague instructions. So use precise numbers, exact times and dates, specific places, and names of persons. Leave no room for doubt in their minds.

Principle: As we've just seen in the previous chapter, Aspies' brains are wired to literally interpret another person's words. You can't change their basic brain circuitry, but you can help them change how they perceive things. You can make it easier—both on you and for them—by keeping instructions or discourse simple, exact, and well-defined. I try to ingrain the mantra "Clarity, specificity, and accountability" in everyone I work with, but this phrase is particularly applicable to Aspies. There's no place for abstractions or generalities. Be exact. Be specific.

L et's look at an example of this principle. Your adult Aspie son, John, has a dentist's appointment tomorrow. Since he lives in his own apartment, doesn't drive, and the van for the disabled doesn't go anywhere near his dentist's office, you'll be providing the transportation. As you start to make the arrangements for the trip, you want to make sure that there are no misunderstandings. So you phone (or e-mail or text) John and say, "John, I'm going to pick you up tomorrow morning around 10 to take you to your appointment. Please make sure you have everything you need."

Guess what? You just messed up big-time. You took too much for granted. The Aspie brain has a hard time processing vague instructions like those. The anxiety begins to kick in immediately.

Imagine you're an Aspie. Here's what John thought when he got that message. "What appointment is he talking about? What does he mean by 'everything I need'? What exact time is he coming? 'Around 10' could be anytime. My brain's not fast enough to process all of this information. I'm not even sure where I'm going. What time will I be back? Do I need to pack my food? Bring a change of clothes? How can I know what 'everything I need' is if I don't even know what time I'm coming back?

Here are the instructions you should have given to John, which would have been much easier for his brain to process: "Please meet me downstairs in front of your apartment building tomorrow morning at 10:15 so I can drive you to your scheduled appointment with the dentist. Make sure you have your ID card and your medical insurance card. When we are finished with the appointment, which should take approximately one hour, I will drive you back to your apartment."

The upside to Aspies taking everything so literally is that specifics work really well with them. They prefer things in black-and-white, and they like explicit instructions and exact numbers. They don't want to have to try to figure out anything. Their anxiety levels soar when you leave it up to them to figure out exactly what it is you'd like them to do, especially if you give them too much leeway and choice. So make it easy on the Aspie and yourself. Be specific.

Action Plan: This one is straightforward. Just say what you mean and mean what you say. Be as specific as possible with numbers, times, dates, locations, colors—you name it. Don't be vague. Be exact. Even as you try to educate Aspies on how the instructions they'll hear in the real world might be open to misinterpretation, you should concentrate on being as clear as you can. Encourage them to ask for specifics if there's the slightest doubt in their minds.

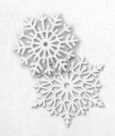

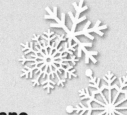

Tip from ESE Teacher Pati Fizzano

It isn't always easy for Aspies to understand and digest what's being asked of them. A teacher may tell an Aspie to do something, and even if the Aspie parrots back the teacher's exact words, it still doesn't mean he truly grasped what the teacher said. Many teachers become frustrated by this. When you're dealing with Aspies, you need a lot of patience and kindness. Getting them to feel comfortable in the classroom can be a challenge. They're shy, and they don't like being the center of attention or being called on in class.

In the world of "Asper Time" (meaning, it can take longer to explain directions for doing something to an Aspie than a non-Aspie), we encourage our teachers to pause after giving an instruction and then have the student repeat the instructions back to them and explain exactly what the instructions are. This ensures that the student understands what's been said. Parents should do this too. If the instruction contains more than one or two steps, they may even want to have the child write it down.

Thought from Rebecca Reitman

Everyone expects the Aspie to be specific, but many of the people in our circle are not always specific enough with *us*. A lot of people who work with Aspies could benefit from reading this chapter.

Aspies need to be trained to repeat a question if they're not sure what's being said to them. Sometimes the tone of someone's voice will throw me off. If their tone gets louder, or if they start to talk faster, I may have a hard time understanding what they're trying to tell me.

Aspies are much more likely to listen to what you are saying if you speak in a gentle tone. If someone is screaming or sounds aggressive, the Aspie is pretty much guaranteed to tune out. We're much more receptive if you respect our hypersensitivity.

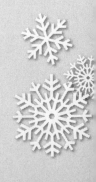

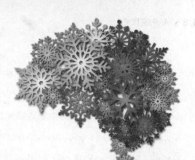

16 PREVENTING OVERWHELM: BREAKING DOWN BIG JOBS INTO SMALLER TASKS

Baby steps!
All I have to do is take
one little step at a time and
I can do anything.

—*Bob Wiley (Bill Murray) in* What About Bob?

Helpful Hint: A task or job with many steps can intimidate Aspies. The prospect of having to complete a huge job can overwhelm them, leading to inaction, anxiety, or even a meltdown. The Aspertool is to break down that big task into mini-tasks— a process called chunking.

Principle: Overwhelm Aspies and you are dooming them to failure. A job that entails multiple steps, even if it does not seem like a big job to you, can seem almost insurmountable to an Aspie. Their brains can't rapidly assimilate all of the different steps needed. They see it as something involving multiple transitions. To enable an Aspie to complete a job, take it one step at a time. Adding steps incrementally will build in the Aspie the confidence necessary to complete the task.

In the movie *What About Bob?*, there's a scene where the psychiatrist, played by Richard Dreyfuss, shows his patient Bob, played by Bill Murray, a "ground-breaking" new book titled *Baby Steps*. Dreyfuss haughtily tells his patient: "It's about setting small reasonable goals for yourself. One tiny step at a time. For instance, when you leave this office, don't think about everything you have to do to get out of building. Just think about what you have to do to get out of this room. When you get to the hall, deal with the hall."

The concept is alluring to Bob, who walks through the office and out the door, chanting, "Baby steps. Baby steps. Oh boy. Baby steps." He exits the office, then pokes his head back in and exclaims, "It works!" Delighted, he says, "Baby steps! All I have to do is take one little step at a time and I can do anything."

It's true. Baby steps work. Breaking a big job up into tinier chunks keeps the Aspie from getting overwhelmed. Take chores, for instance. Telling an Aspie (or any kid), "Your room's a disaster. Clean it up right now!" won't work. You've got to break down what seems to her a Herculean task into smaller, discrete steps so it won't be so daunting. "First, pick up your dirty clothes and put them in the hamper. Then make your bed. Call me when those two jobs are done." It would be best, of course, to schedule in routines as much as possible, but when routines change, chunking is a way to make things manageable.

For example, Andy, the owner of a small construction company, was working with his somewhat autistic stepson Tony on a home renovation. They had to pull up a very big tile floor. Andy had worked on projects with his stepson before and knew from experience that Tony knew how to remove individual tiles with the type of impact drill known as a mini-jackhammer (wearing protective earmuffs to shut out the noise—essential for anyone and especially an Aspie). But Andy made the mistake of telling Tony to take up the *whole* floor. He told Tony to come and get him when the job was done in its entirety, and then he went outside to work on another part of the house.

The thought of taking up the *whole* floor overwhelmed Tony. He started pacing. He walked around in circles. He twitched. Basically, he had an extreme anxiety attack.

When Andy came back to check on his stepson an hour later, he was stunned to see that not a single tile had been removed. Realizing they were now behind schedule, Andy blew his top, which practically sent Tony into a full-blown meltdown.

It took Andy two years to learn how to work with his stepson. Now he knows how to leverage the philosophy of chunking. Here's how the same scenario plays out these days:

"Tony, I know you know how to work the jackhammer and take up tiles. Do you see these four tiles right here? You take them up, put them in a nice pile over there, and when you're done, come get me." Andy goes outside. Twenty minutes later, Tony comes out with a big smile, brings Andy back inside, and shows him that he has completed the task.

Andy says, "Good job, Tony. Now, can you take up those six tiles over here?" Tony smiles and takes up six more tiles as Andy works outside. When that chunk of the job is done, he goes outside to get Andy again. By the end of the day Tony is taking up twelve tiles at a time, has pulled up the entire floor, and is beaming with joy at having performed the job with excellence. He's put in a productive day's work, with results as good as any professional could have achieved.

Action Plan: A large task will overwhelm an Aspie and become a self-fulfilling prophecy of failure if you don't show her how to do it one step at a time. Ask, "What am I trying to accomplish?" The answer is not that you're trying to get the job done the fastest way, but that you're trying to do it the best way, with the best results, and in a manner that works for the Aspie. Remember, Rome wasn't built in a day.[21] Properly harnessing the Aspie's abilities will lead to a mutually beneficial situation where the work will get done with excellence, and the Aspie will gain self-esteem for a job well done. And self-esteem is a great reward for Aspies for trumping the challenges they encounter each day.

21 James Clear, who writes about using behavioral science to master your habits, is fond of saying, "Rome wasn't built in a day, but they were laying bricks every hour. Actually Rome is just the result, the bricks are the system. The system is greater than the goal. Focusing on your habits is more important than worrying about your outcomes....[L]aying brick is not a fantastic amount of work. It's not a grand feat of strength or stamina or intelligence. But laying a brick every day, year after year? That's how you build an empire."

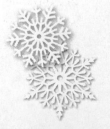

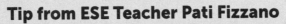

Tip from ESE Teacher Pati Fizzano

Project assignments are a source of anxiety for Aspies. If we don't break a project down by *chunking it into smaller components*, it won't get done. For example, a project for the science fair project may be due in six weeks. After we give the initial instructions, we ask the students to bring in specific parts of the project over the six-week span. By the last week, all that's left to do are the final touches. Chunking this type of assignment helps Aspies stay focused and also gives the teachers the opportunity to provide feedback each week to make sure the students are doing the project correctly.

Thought from Rebecca Reitman

When I was in college—which was before I knew I had Asperger's—I sometimes used chunking, but more often used procrastination-based activities to accomplish my work. Toward the end, I definitely didn't chunk but worked endless hours on my math coursework, which was extremely frustrating. Sometimes if the material, or the way the teacher presented it, was too confusing I would just faze out or accomplish other things rather than listening. Luckily, I had great tutors.

I can tell you from experience that chunking is absolutely necessary when Aspies are facing a large project or task. They need to have the project put into smaller parts, perhaps even slivers or slices. The smaller the slice, the easier it is to deal with when asking for help.

17 SETTING GOALS

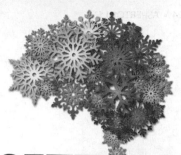

Most impossible goals can
be met simply by breaking them
down into bite-size chunks, writing
them down, believing them, and
then going full speed ahead
as if they were routine.

— Don Lancaster

Arriving at one goal is
the starting point
to another.

— John Dewey

Helpful Hint: It's important to set goals for an Aspie. Aspies live by goals; they need to achieve. However, Aspies cannot be changed overnight. The goals set for them must be met one by one.

T he adage "parents know what's best for their child" usually holds true. The exception is when the parents of an Aspie create a long list of ambitious goals for their child. An Aspie cannot be changed overnight. When parents set goals for an Aspie, they should do so incrementally. Parents should write down every change or goal they'd like for their children, then order them by importance. They should discuss the goals with their children and be sure that everyone agrees on the importance of each goal. When everyone is on the same page, then they can set the rules, rewards, and consequences for each goal.

When Pati first began working with Rebecca a year or two ago, she knew we needed to take small steps to reach all the goals we had—for Rebecca and for our family as well. Pati asked each of us to identify what we wanted to accomplish and to rank each item on the list by importance. My priority was to have more positive communication with Rebecca each day. So together with Pati, we established the rule that Rebecca and I would phone each other once a day. All conversation had to be positive, and whoever dialed the other would be the one to exit the call by saying something nice. Each call was to last at least five minutes but not more than fifteen. The rule was specific, with rewards and consequences set in place. This seemingly simple goal was anything but—it took eight months to achieve it to the satisfaction of both Rebecca and me. But calling me on the phone now comes naturally to Rebecca.

A family goal was to have a monthly get-together. To achieve this goal, we set aside one day a month for having a family meal and playing some board games. Other goals included getting Rebecca more involved socially, bringing her to the middle school to tutor, and attending family get-togethers with less reluctance. We crossed them off the list one by one.

If we had tried to reach all our goals at once, or if we had told Rebecca about all of the items on the list as we started them, she'd have thought we were overloading her and we'd never have achieved even one of the goals.

Action Plan: Parents or caring third parties must realize they can't tackle all their goals for their Aspies at once. Introduce goals gradually, and master each one before going on to the next. If you try to move through the goals too quickly or introduce them all at once, you will end up with an epic fail. Take your time working with your child to achieve your goals and his goals. Let him believe he's controlling his life. Moving at a deliberate pace on something so important frustrates many parents. Just remember: One step at a time, and pick your battles carefully.

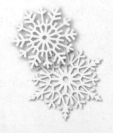

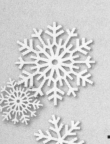

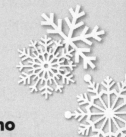

Tip from ESE Teacher Pati Fizzano

When we set goals on the Aspie's Individualized Education Program (IEP) at school, we never set more than four. If we overload Aspies with goals, they may shut down on us.

Communication is always one of the key IEP goals. One example is "pragmatic language," which refers to the art of conversation (taking turns speaking, staying on topic, or showing interest in what others are saying). The school's speech pathologist will also work on prosody, which refers to the tone or volume of someone's voice or how fast he talks.

Another IEP goal is fluency in reading. Many of our Aspie students love to read but have a hard time comprehending what they're reading. We track students to determine if they're achieving their reading goals:

1. During every marking period (report card time), we update their goal sheets.

2. We "grade" them as no progress, some progress, almost mastered, or mastered.

3. We review their goals four times in an IEP year.

4. Once the Aspie masters a goal, we introduce a new goal for him.

It's not a good idea to make achieving goals a game. Aspies take their goals too seriously. If you make it a game, they won't know if you're serious about the goals or not, and you'll lose them.

Thought from Rebecca Reitman

Don't expect the Aspie to do everything at once. Overloading an Aspie can lead to an immediate meltdown.

Even after an Aspie achieves a goal or masters a task, the parent should not cross it out of his journal. The Aspie may always have a "relapse." The parent can check it off, but it's a good idea to keep a list of mastered goals.

If the Aspie is not an only child, he should see that his siblings have goals too. The siblings' goals need to be made obvious to the Aspie to ensure he doesn't feel different from the other children. As my dad says, "What's good for the goose is good for the gander."

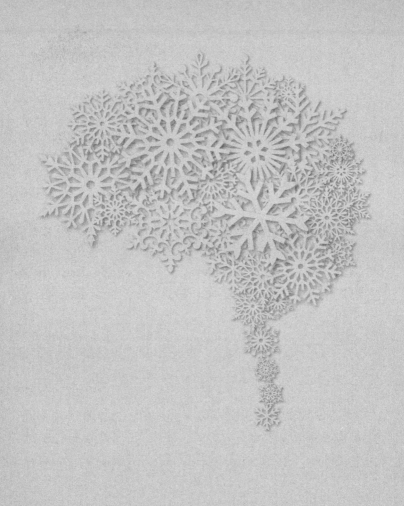

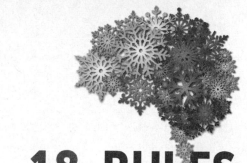

18 RULES, REWARDS, AND CONSEQUENCES

> Reward and punishment are
> the only motives to a rational creature:
> these are the spur and reins whereby
> all mankind are set on
> work, and guided.
>
> *—John Locke*

Helpful Hint: Making rules and backing them up is a good way to effect changes in behavior. Just remember: rules, rewards, and consequences must be fair and apply to all parties, not just the Aspie. The concept of fairness is important to everyone but is of extreme importance to the Aspie. You must be consistent. Consistency is a valuable Aspertool.

Principle: A system of rules, enforced through consequences and rewards, constitutes the most fundamental method of behavior modification for an individual as well as society as a whole. And as with many of the issues discussed in this book, it is something that is even more applicable to Aspies. To bring about positive changes in your Aspie's behavior, you must have rules and enforce them through rewards and consequences. If your Aspie disobeys a rule, she needs a consequence—a punishment or effectively negative reinforcement geared to the Aspie, with a positive twist—delivered in a timely fashion. If she follows a rule consistently, the Aspie should be rewarded; positive reinforcement goes a long way. Aspies consider praise to be one of the highest rewards.

Just as Aspies have hyper-senses, they also have hyper-adherence to rules. Once a rule is made and enforced, an Aspie will hardly ever break it. But the Aspie wants to see that you're obeying the rule as well. What's good for the goose is good for the gander. It's only fair. If you're a parent of three kids—an Aspie and two neurotypical siblings—the rules have to apply to all three kids. And you too. The whole family has to obey the rules. To the Aspie, that's justice.

Simple enough—all parties play by the same rules. The parent (or teacher, therapist, or tutor) has to make sure there are consequences if *you* break the rule. "Do as I say, not as I do" doesn't apply here. But keep in mind the Aspie's essential need for clarity, specificity, and accountability, as well as her taking words literally, because it means you'll be putting yourself on trial every day.

For example, the following e-mail is about a "well-intentioned parent" failing to obey the rules. I broke a rule I'd made for Rebecca. And when she pointed out that I'd broken the rule, I gave her words a curt dismissal. Another instance of my super-busy self being the proverbial bull in the china shop, not only being wrong but unthinkingly doing damage on several fronts.

Subject: Rules work both ways
From: Hackie
To: Rebecca

Dear Rebecca,

Let me start off by saying you're right—it has taken me a long time to learn certain lessons, one being the lesson about rules working both ways.

In our conversation earlier today, you said you were surprised that my e-mail included a one-word reference to the organization helping us with the attempted theft of your ID. That was a keen observation. But I replied in a dismissive manner. I want to apologize for that.

You and I are similar in that we both work better with rules than with thinking through an exception to everything. My rule has been for you not to share any confidential information unless absolutely necessary. When I sent out the group e-mail, even though I didn't include any confidential information, it was still wrong of me to mention anything about the specific name.

I did this because I wanted your independent living facility coaches to know there were several attempted fraud and identity theft incidents directed at you. I thought if they were aware of that, they'd keep their eyes and ears open. I was trying to bring this to their attention without providing any real details. Still, what I did was not consistent with what I've been advising you.

When you pointed this out, I should have paused, weighed what you were saying, and given you a thoughtful response. Instead, I reacted in a knee-jerk way and responded—curtly but politely—that the e-mail contained no confidential material.

The rule, which you stated very clearly, is that no information about anything confidential should be included in such a group e-mail. I broke that rule.

These days, as I write the book about Aspies, I find myself thinking more and more about situations like this. Often, something that happened in the past comes back to me and then, all this time later, I'm finally able to understand what was going on back then. Maybe the book should have a chapter on how rules work both ways.

I hope the above makes some sense. Again, I'm so very sorry for my dismissive response.

Love, Dad

I include this e-mail not just to show how terrible I felt (feeling terrible after the fact is a feeling many of us "well-intentioned parents" know all too well) but because it exemplifies another tool: admitting when you're wrong. Aspies relish *mea culpas*, especially those from their parents.

For an Aspie, life is a constant struggle to meet the expectations of a parent, teacher, boss, or even society. Few things are more *demoralizing* to Aspies than when they finally *do it right,* not only is it not appreciated but it gets thrown in their faces that the neurotypical parent or sibling is *allowed* to break the rules with no consequences. That's not fair. Justice has not been served. And justice, fairness, and truth are three important concepts to Aspies, as they should be to all of us.

Explain What They Did Wrong

Before you correct an Aspie for doing something wrong, ask if she knows what she did wrong and, more important, why it was wrong. If she doesn't know, take the time to explain it. Calmly. Patiently. Pleasantly. Admonishing the Aspie in a raised voice only hurts her brain because of her hypersensitive hearing, and the situation will escalate. Then go into your Aspertoolbox for rules and consequences to prevent the action or behavior from recurring. It is a teachable moment.

Aspies get frustrated by the neurotypical's lack of understanding of how their brains work and why they do what they do. Many times they cannot express it in words. Sometimes they have the best intentions to behave appropriately, but they can't figure out how to do so. Even when they do figure it out, they can't get the words out fast enough. When Aspies fail in their attempt to use logic and other pathways in their brains to modify their behavior positively, it can be a profound disappointment, not just to the Aspie but to all concerned.

Choose the Consequence Carefully— Minimize Collateral Damage

Principle: After telling your Aspie that it's rude to raise one's voice during a discussion, you made a rule about it (which you also have to obey). Now choose the consequence . . . carefully. In setting the punishment, try to minimize collateral damage— unintended negative consequences to "innocent bystanders."

An example will help illustrate this principle. It's Saturday morning. You're waiting in front of the apartment building where Tim, your twenty-three-year-old Aspie, lives. Tim was supposed to meet you downstairs at exactly eleven o'clock so you could drive him to his piano lesson. But just like last Saturday and the Saturday before that and the Saturday before that, he's running about twenty minutes late.

You know you can rectify the situation with a rule and the proper consequence. If Tim were trying to catch a bus and missed it, the bus would leave without him. So that could be the consequence: you drive away after a grace period of five or ten minutes. (You would clearly communicate this consequence to Tim ahead of time.) After you drove away once or twice, Tim would figure out how to be on time (assuming he enjoys his piano lesson). Of course, keep in mind the downsides of this consequence.

- **Tim misses a positive structured activity.**
- **The piano teacher suffers unintended collateral damage.**
- **You have to pay for a lesson that never took place.**

Watch out for unintended negative consequences. You don't want to make the consequence something that detracts from your Aspie's socialization, for example, Tim can't attend his Aspie group meet-up or go on his weekly walk with his friends. But you could factor in the Aspie's reluctance to be with other people, and make the consequence Tim's mandatory attendance at a family event he'd prefer to avoid.

You decide that whenever Tim is late, the consequence would be missing his favorite weekly TV show and spending that time reading or engaging in a social activity. Once that consequence was established, Tim was late only one more time; now he's always punctual. Problem solved through an Aspertool.

Action Plan: View the consequence through Aspies' eyes. It has to be something they'd consider a punishment. Ideally, it would relate to the rule that was broken, but that's not always practical. I think of the consequence not so much as a punishment but as an opportunity to have Aspies do something that's good for them but that they prefer not to do. In fact, once they try it, they might actually come to like it. Turn a negative into a positive.

A Reward Should Be Something They Want, Not What You Want

Principle: Your Aspie is following a rule to the letter, and you want that positive behavior to continue. The Aspertool is to reward good behavior with something the recipient really wants and appreciates. Through *observation* you'll need to figure out the positive things your Aspie really enjoys. It can be an activity, a food, a new pair of sneakers . . . you name it. Or let the Aspie name it. Then offer that as a reward if she follows the rules. Just be sure it's something the Aspie wants, not what you want. Ideally, it should be a reward with positive value.

For example, Frank, an adult Aspie, has been on time for his job for two weeks straight. You want to buy him some reading material as positive reinforcement. You know what Frank likes to read because you've observed him. So do you buy him a book on some nutritious diet because it'd be good for his health? How about a copy of *Time* so he can keep up on current events? No, you surprise Frank with what he really wants: a new comic book featuring his favorite Marvel superhero. The reward should be wonderful *as seen through Frank's eyes,* as long as it's not a negative thing. A Marvel comic might not be your cup of tea, but Frank enjoys them and admires the values espoused by his superheroes. It makes him happy, which will encourage continued positive behavior.

Action Plan: *Observe* your Aspie so you know what she
really enjoys and which rewards she'd appreciate. Better yet, ask
your Aspie what she enjoys (preferably when you're just making
conversation, not when it's time for the reward). It's a good topic
of conversation, and you often learn something you didn't know
about her. Just make sure what she enjoys is something positive.
Once you've come up with some potential rewards, start looking
for positive behaviors that are worthy of these rewards. *Parents
can get so busy looking for negative behaviors to punish that they
don't take the time to find good behavior patterns that deserve to
be rewarded.* Positive reinforcement is an underused Aspertool.
Use it! Get positive! Have fun with this!

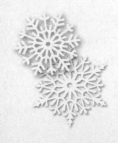

Tip from ESE Teacher Pati Fizzano

Aspies learn best when their school environment is highly structured. One way I structure my classes is through a system of rules based on reward points and fines. For good behavior, students get reward points; for negative behavior, such as bullying, pushing, hitting, or not completing their homework, they're assessed fines. Reward points are added to the student's daily planner each day by a teacher. Fines are paid each Friday. A chart on the wall displays a running total of everyone's points. Points can be redeemed for time playing board games or treats. At the end of the semester we tally up the points for special end-of-the-year rewards, such as a trip to a restaurant or an auction of items the students like.

A reward can never be taken away from a student once they've earned it. To help my students better understand the concept of fines, I explain that if you deposited $100 from your paycheck into your bank account on Monday, then got a $15 parking ticket on Wednesday, you'd pay the fine with money from your bank account. But your employer didn't take away any money from your paycheck. The fine was for bad judgment, and now you have to pay the fine.

The system has worked with all my students, especially one boy who was being particularly difficult. This boy had previously attended other middle schools, where he was constantly receiving detention, before coming to us in eighth grade. The concept of reward points clicked with him. He started to flourish and attained high grades.

Thought from Rebecca Reitman

I am a rule follower! Everyone involved must agree to the rules. It truly frustrates me when others break rules and receive no consequences. If a rule is unfair and I cannot agree to it, I call that an "Aspie Code." Aspies usually tell the truth, but if they have to deal with an Aspie Code, they will adjust the rule and find ways around it.

Rewards motivate Aspies to do something, especially if it's something they don't really want to do. A reward does not need to be of a monetary value. Praise is one of the best motivators for me. And a consequence must fit the crime, or else it won't make sense to an Aspie.

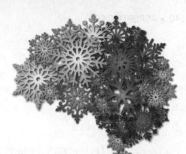

19 CHECKLISTS: THE INDISPENSABLE TOOL

Good checklists are easy to use
even in the most difficult situations.
They do not try to spell out everything.
They provide reminders of only the
most important steps—the ones that even
the highly skilled professional using
them could miss. Good checklists
are, above all, practical.

—*Atul Gawande,* The Checklist Manifesto:
How to Get Things Right

Helpful Hint: All of us use checklists now and then, but for Aspies, checklists are indispensable. A simple checklist will help them make sure they did all their tasks when they were supposed to. It can remind them what to eat for breakfast or what to wear. It can relieve much of their anxiety about appointments, will help them be on time, and will even help them become more independent. Once they see that a task is checked off, they can relax knowing it's been accomplished. They don't have to stress over whether they remembered to do it as they're rushing out the door. A good checklist can at times be a partial substitute for an Aspie's lack of executive function.

Principle: The mundane details of daily living that neurotypicals sleepwalk through are daunting to the poor Aspie: getting up on time, remembering to brush his teeth, take a shower, put on clean underwear, get dressed, eat a good breakfast, and bring everything he'll need for the day ahead. Getting out the door. In addition to lacking the overall *executive functioning*[22] to perform this list of daily chores, moving from each one requires a *transition*, and as we've already seen, transitions can overwhelm Aspies. Now stir in their anxiety, the pressure to be on time, and the constant interruptions that besiege all of us, and you have a recipe for failure. The Aspie might just decide that rather than walk out the door, it's easier to go back to the undemanding environment of his bedroom.

What can give them the confidence of knowing that as they walk out the door, they have not forgotten something yet again? What can help them see not the formidability of one big, overwhelming task but a series of smaller accomplishable tasks? Answer: A checklist, the easy-to-create tool that will reduce Aspies' anxiety and make their day run smoothly. All they need is a piece of paper and a pen. This simple document will constantly change, but at any one point in time it is fixed, specific, and in order, just the way an Aspie likes. The checklist makes the Aspie's daily activities more predictable and therefore less stressful and helps the Aspie navigate each day's landscape more efficiently.

Like any change to Aspies' environments, don't expect your Aspie to welcome the idea of the checklist at first. Introduce it to his routine gradually. Once the checklist becomes part of his beloved routine, he'll come to embrace it. It will be like a dependable guide dog that helps him keep up with the transitions of each day and prevents him from feeling overwhelmed or panicked. Just remember, don't try to establish the entire checklist at once. Baby steps! Chunking, in effect.

When Aspies look at the checklist and see that every item has been checked off, they'll gain confidence from that reassuring visual. And out the door they'll go with a "Whew!" and a smile, instead of worrying, "What did I forget this time?"

Even after the Aspie embraces this Aspertool, someone—a parent, a teacher, a caring third party, or even one of the Aspie's friends—will still have to check up on him regularly to make sure he's following the checklist. That someone is part of the circle of those entrusted to ensure that the checklist is being completed. All the members of the circle must do their part.

As Aspies learn how to add items to the checklist, their independence will be maximized. That's the goal. Some (but not most) Aspies evolve so that they can check on themselves and no longer need a third party to do that.

Imagine you're an Aspie. You know you have to be at the event taking place across the street in ten minutes. Just as you get ready to leave your apartment, a barrage of questions comes rushing to your brain. "Do I have everything? Am I dressed properly? Do I have my medications with me? Do I have my directions to the meeting room? What am I forgetting?" A quick glance at the checklist you prepared the night before reminds you of everything you need to do and bring. You breathe a sigh of relief, and out the door you go.

We all need tools to help us remember everything we need to. (I've never figured out exactly what my "label" is, but I feel that same type of "Do I have everything?" anxiety each time I go through airport security. And there have been times when I started walking to the gate from the security area, only to realize I'd forgotten my laptop computer!) But for the Aspie that need is magnified. As with all Aspertools, the key is getting Aspies to accept the methods that will maximize their independence long after we are gone. A checklist is a part of a system of dependable things that will reduce the need for helicopter parents so that the Aspie can have a fulfilling, safe, productive life and an independent existence. This is what everyone in the Aspie circle is after. However, anyone in the circle—teacher, coach, student, parent, friend—can break it by neglecting his duty, to the detriment of the student.

In many schools the Aspies use a checklist-like tool, a simple homework planner to write down their daily assignments. The teacher checks them every so often to make sure the Aspies are writing down the correct assignments. If they are, they get a reward; if not, they get a fine or another consequence. The student then takes the planner home and a parent checks the work and signs off on it. This is how the circle works with the school planner.

For example, an eighth-grade Aspie named Daniel created his checklist of assignments with the help of his ESE teacher and left school confident that he was all set to take care of his homework. At home, however, he became confused with his assignments, and his mother neglected to go over his work and check off the items on his planner. Daniel came to school the next day without having completed his tasks and therefore received a fine—a deduction of the points he'd accrued for all his positive activities, points he could turn in for prizes. This negative cycle repeated itself for a week. The fines piled up. The teacher called Daniel's mom to discuss it. It turns out that the harried mother had been neglecting her role in the circle.

This is not unusual. Parents are often the ones who break the circle. Many parents say to themselves, "Oh, I'll sign the checklist later . . ." but forget to do it. Unfortunately, when that happens, the student suffers the consequences. Then the teacher feels bad because he has to "fine" the Aspie student.

Ultimately, the checklist should be the Aspies' responsibility, an independent goal for them to accomplish without others checking on them. But when I asked Daniel's ESE teacher, who specializes in Asperger's, how many of her eighth-graders were creating their checklists independently, her answer was only two of the eleven students.

Action Plan: Make sure your Aspie gets the help he needs to create a checklist and keep it current. Individuals in the "circle" should know their role and their schedule for checking on the Aspie. Checklists will keep the individual Aspie from being overwhelmed by the activities of daily living. The checklist—finite, tangible, specific—is easy to implement. Best of all, it works. All in all, it's one of the most effective Aspertools.

---

22 Executive function (also known as cognitive control and supervisory attentional system) is an umbrella term for the management (regulation, control) of cognitive processes, including working memory, reasoning, task flexibility, and problem solving, as well as planning and execution.

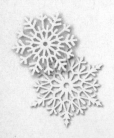

Tip from ESE teacher Pati Fizzano

A checklist should be designed for Aspies. For younger children, the parents can create a "picture checklist" of what they need to do and tack it to a wall. For instance, a checklist in the bathroom would show pictures of a toothbrush, comb, and so on.

In school the checklist is mandatory. We begin in sixth grade with the "circle of checklist." The circle consists of the student, the teacher, and the parent. Students write down the assignment in their journals, the teacher signs the journals to indicate it was done, and the parents check their children's journals and sign it. If one of the parties in the checklist circle doesn't sign the journal, you can be assured the homework will not be done.

Mastering the checklist takes a good two and a half years, but at the end of that time students are well trained. During eighth grade, I move away from the checklist circle and give each student a homework planner book, the kind many adults use in their daily lives. The planner reminds students what they have to do in terms of completing their homework, studying for tests, and finishing projects. For Aspies it also reinforces the notion that they must complete their work at home with guidance from their parents. This gives my Aspie students a taste of what high school is like, although I still monitor them. By the time my students have finished eighth grade, I know they're ready for high school. The checklist has helped them become more independent.

Last year I had a very disorganized student. Alex was never ready for math class, which frustrated his math teacher. Even when he saw the other kids laying out their supplies, he wouldn't do it. The teacher would say, "Alex, do I have to tell you *every day* to have your pencil, your book, and your calculator out on your desk?" Finally I wrote out a mini-checklist on an index card: Pencil. Book. Calculator. I taped it to his desk. We never had an issue with Alex again.

Adult Aspies have learned to use their smartphones as a checklist-like tool. Recently I was sitting with two Aspies at a dinner party. Both of their phones chimed within seconds of each other. The first Aspie asked, "What is that a reminder for?"

"To take my pills," the second answered. "And your reminder is for . . .?"

"That I need to feed my fish," the first said.

Thought from Rebecca Reitman

Checklists need to be established for everything from the time the Aspie wakes up to the time he goes to bed. There should be one for the morning routine, one for school, and one for the evening routines. Each checklist should include, in particular, the things that don't come natural to Aspies, or the tasks they don't like doing. The simpler the better is the best rule for these, keeping in mind the acronym KISS: Keep It Simple, Stupid.

I use checklists developed by my coach. Most of the time I print the sheets out weekly and put an X next to the completed tasks. I let Rosalie know about the morning checklist completion, for the most part, via e-mail. However, she can always see my lists and my progress on the lists when she comes to my apartment.

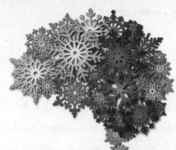

20 TIME MANAGEMENT: TOOLS FOR GETTING YOUR ASPIE TO BE ON TIME

How did it get so late so soon?
It's night before it's afternoon.
December is here before it's June.
My goodness how the time has flewn.
How did it get so late so soon?

— *Dr. Seuss*

Helpful Hint: Time management is difficult for most of us, but especially Aspies. They need help to stay on schedule. That help can come in the form of Aspertools. A system of rules, rewards, and consequences will encourage the Aspie to be punctual. Another Aspertool, a simple checklist, can help relieve the anxiety that often hinders an Aspie trying to be on schedule.

Principle: Time is our most precious resource. When I think how God gives us only a certain amount of time on this planet, and how much of it we squander, it motivates me to get as much done each day as I can. As my longtime friend, the great sports handicapper Lem Banker, once put it to me, "God made all of us equal. He gives every one of us twenty-four hours each day. What we do with those twenty-four hours is up to each of us."

To a neurotypical, time is a simple unit—a second is 1/60 of a minute, a minute is 1/60 of an hour, an hour is 1/24 of a day. But to Aspies, time is yet another pathway in the convoluted maze of activities they navigate every day. Not only do they have to remember what tasks to do hour by hour throughout the day, but also they have to remember the order in which to do those tasks, which ones are higher priority, as well as "down-to-the-minute time assignments" for each one. The world they live in is an exact, demanding, and unforgiving one. It's hard for them to chunk it out.

Because Aspies tend to have poor *executive function*, they don't fare well at the little details that neurotypicals take for granted, such as prioritizing to-dos, assigning a proper sequence to their tasks, and keeping on schedule. This is why *routine* is so important to Aspies. Being in a good routine reduces their need to continually connect all the dots of daily living, a task that their circuitry is ill-equipped to handle. A routine helps them not to have to reinvent the wheel.

For example, George is a fourteen-year-old Aspie with a high degree of anxiety. Although he's an honor student, a lot of his anxiety is related to attending school. As a result, he started getting to school at least a half hour late every day. This went on for weeks. Finally Pati called George's mother in for a meeting. The mom said she had tried everything to get George to be on time for school. From her experience, Pati sensed that George was "playing" his mom.

To address the situation, Pati "pulled out" several tools from her Aspertoolbox. First, she had George and his mom create a *checklist* of all the things he needed to do each morning before leaving the house. Then came the *rule*. From having *observed* George, Pati knew that he liked leaving school the very second the final bell rang. So Pati established the *rule* that if George was not at school at 8 AM sharp, even thirty seconds late, he'd suffer the *consequences* for breaking the rule. And the consequence was that for every minute George was late to school in the morning, he'd be required to stay after school for the exact same amount of time.

The next day George was twelve minutes late, so he had to stay twelve minutes after school. Every one of those twelve minutes George had to stay after the final bell was sheer torture. Pati's consequence worked. George didn't repeat his mistake again. He came to school on time every day. His mother can't believe that a single, simple Aspertool could make such a difference in her son as well as her mornings.

Another illustration of this principle is something from Rebecca. Every Friday at 11 AM, Rebecca has a workout scheduled with her trainer, Ian Pyka, in Coral Springs, about twenty minutes away. I'd swing by her independent living facility at 10:15 AM to drive her there. (I'd built in a fifteen-minute buffer to allow for traffic and the fact that Rebecca was habitually running about fifteen minutes behind.) Rebecca always had a different excuse for being behind schedule. She had to go to the bathroom. She had to pack her lunch. She hadn't slept well the night before due to anxiety. I got fed up with having to wait for her every time and messing up Ian's schedule.

I finally decided it was time for the two of us to get to the bottom of Rebecca's habitual lateness. We used our Aspertools. After observing a typical morning for Rebecca, we determined it was a combination of poor *executive function* and her *anxiety* over whether she had everything she needed when it was time to walk out the door. Next, we established the *rule* that she would do as much preparation as she could the night before. Then Rebecca and her coach created a *checklist*, which would eliminate the panic she often felt, fearing that, as I was waiting, she'd forgotten her meds, her food, her water, or something else. The checklist scheduled all her "getting ready tasks" down to the minute. With the help of all these tools, Rebecca is now on time for her workout with Ian every week.

Action Plan: When you get frustrated because your Aspie is always running late, you need to help her compensate for her inherent difficulty with time management and her lack of executive function. Use all the tools at your disposal to motivate her to be punctual. Help her to create a trusted checklist and incorporate it into her daily routine, including down-to-the-minute "time assignments." Make sure she has enough time to accomplish the tasks she must perform to be on time.

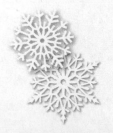

Tip from ESE Teacher Pati Fizzano

Time management may be difficult for an Aspie. One of my time management tips is to have Aspies set their cell phone timers for five minutes earlier than the pick-up time. For example, if you plan on picking your Aspie up at 10 AM, tell her to set the alarm at 9:55 AM. When the alarm goes off, let your Aspie know to STOP what she is doing, DROP everything, and LEAVE. This will make her on time.

Another Aspertool is to have a consequence for lateness. Aspies try very hard not to break rules or suffer consequences.

Thought from Rebecca Reitman

These days my father picks me up at 10:16 every Friday morning. I'm sure you're wondering, "Why 10:16? Why not 10:15?" The reason is that sixteen is a square number. I find that square root numbers are easier for me to remember. As Pati says, "Aspies love patterns; in fact, they can get obsessed with them. For example, squares [square root numbers] are a pattern."

It's really cool when the hour and the minutes separately are both square numbers. It's even cooler when the hour squared = the minute. And it's really awesome when the time is actually a perfect square (without the colon).

As you can see, I use my mathematical obsession to my advantage. I am great with numbers, and it's easier for me to remember things in terms of special numbers or other interests.

Anyway, I am still sometimes late but not as often as before. I usually wish that the pick-up time was thirty minutes later.

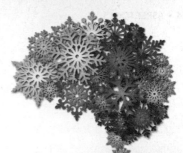

21 OVERLAPPING CONDITIONS

> For strange effects and
> extraordinary combinations we
> must go to life itself, which is always
> far more daring than any effort
> of the imagination.
>
> —*Sir Arthur Conan Doyle*

Helpful Hint: Asperger's syndrome and its various components often occur in combination with other neurological, psychological, and physical disorders. It helps to know something about such overlapping conditions so that you can keep an eye out for any signs of them in your observation of your Aspie. You also want to document as much as possible and have a complete medical summary available. Aspies come in many flavors with many different combinations of related conditions. When you've met one Aspie, you've met one Aspie. Each one is unique.

Principle: It's the rare affliction that does not occur without overlapping, related conditions. This can lead you into countless esoteric chicken-or-the-egg debates. But the important thing is not which condition came first but to make sure you're aware of all the conditions your Aspie must deal with, not because of the labels but because of the interrelationships of all these conditions.

A nxiety plays a major role in any mental or psychological condition you can think of. But in an Aspie, anxiety is magnified to the umpteenth degree. Besides learning to deal with anxiety, you will also need to be on the lookout for obsessive-compulsive disorder (OCD), ADHD, and variations of attention-deficit disorder syndromes, as well as other serious problems like seizure disorders or epilepsy.[23] Related physical disorders such as gastrointestinal disorders and, in some cases, hypersensitivity are within the intestinal system of the Aspie. The key is to know as much as possible about all the related neurological and psychological conditions. I could dazzle you with a bunch of other abbreviations, eponyms, and fancy names, or you could find them with a search engine, just as I did.

Don't let my MD fool you. Just to repeat, I'm not writing this book as a medical professional. Like you, I'm just another "well-intentioned parent" who was once totally clueless but has now ascended to the lofty perch of "less cluelessdom." Of course, it's a lot easier to be less clueless today than back when I was in med school, when learning about a medical condition meant a trip to the graduate stacks at the university library. Now you can get an in-depth explanation of anything by typing a few keywords into your search engine. So you can learn a lot in a little time about any issue that comes up with your Aspie.

Action Plan: Make sure appropriate specialists have fully evaluated your Aspie and that you have in your possession one comprehensive medical summary. You might have to compile it yourself. We doctors used to joke that as everything in medicine got more specialized, specialists knew more and more about less and less until ultimately they knew everything about nothing. That joke is not so far-fetched anymore. Things are so specialized today that the various specialists have a difficult time communicating with one another.

Because of this situation, one of your many tasks is to be the chief interpreter and translator of your Aspie's medical history. Someone has to have a comprehensive copy of the medical records, medications, and medical tests, as well as an overall summary of them. This way, if your Aspie visits a new specialist—psychologist, psychiatrist, neurologist—you can just hand them the medical summary, along with any supporting reports. (This will also come in handy when applying for various programs, accommodations, and services). Doing this forces all concerned parties to be aware of the entire situation and all overlapping conditions. Asperger's syndrome rarely exists in a vacuum. Neither does any other problem for the Aspie or, for that matter, the neurotypical. Nobody gets a pass.

---

23 There are also all kinds of overlapping indications for medications. Some antiseizure meds are also antianxiety meds/sleeping meds/mood changers. Off-label use has opened up what some feel is a harmful Pandora's box and what others hope is a magic bullet. And let's face it; we well-intentioned parents are always seeking magic bullets.

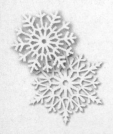

Tip from ESE Teacher Pati Fizzano

Many Aspies have overlapping conditions. When I first meet with a new Aspie student, I review his Individualized Education Program (IEP), which is a guide to help the teachers understand their students and to help the students reach their educational goals. The IEP includes their primary and additional exceptionalities, overlapping conditions, current performance, goal pages, related services, and their accommodations.

Thought from Rebecca Reitman

Aspies can have overlapping *DSM* conditions (conditions recognized by the *Diagnostic and Statistical Manual*) develop before, during, or after they are diagnosed with Asperger's. Sometimes there is a definite cause and effect behind the appearance of post-Aspie diagnosis conditions. For example, an Aspie friend of mine had several other *DSM* conditions. She thought she was fat, and when a male student at our school affirmed her self-image, she acquired an eating disorder and became anorexic. She made sure she kept losing weight. Other *DSM* conditions *are* often diagnosed prior to an Asperger's diagnosis, especially in females, because females hide being an Aspie better than males do.

Parents must know that the social services and assistance provided to their Aspies do not end with high school. They must immediately provide the same documentation to the colleges their children will attend; this way, they can get the services started immediately. It would be good if a general practitioner (GP) or some other qualified professional provides the documentation for you to hand to the colleges' disability services administrators.

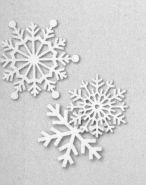

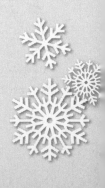

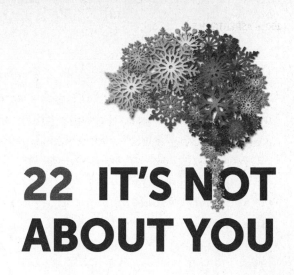

22 IT'S NOT ABOUT YOU

> The merry-go-round
> just goes around.
> I like the roller coaster.
> You get more out of it.
>
> —*Grandmother in* Parenthood

Helpful Hint: Never forget, it's not about you.
It's about your Aspie.

*P*arenthood is one of the great movies about, well, being a parent. In one of my favorite scenes, the grandmother (played by the late Helen Shaw) explains to her grandson Gil (Steve Martin) and his wife, Karen (Mary Steenburgen), the difference between a merry-go-round and a roller coaster.

Grandma: *When I was nineteen, Grandpa took me on a roller coaster.*

Gil (uninterested): *Oh?*

Grandma: *Up. Down. Up. Down. Oh, what a ride.*

Gil (clearly uninterested): *What a great story.*

Grandma: *I always wanted to go again. It was just interesting to me that a ride could make me so frightened, so scared, so sick, so excited, and so thrilled, all together. Some didn't like it. They were on a merry-go-round. But that just goes around. Nothing. I like the roller coaster. You get more out of it.*

The "emotional roller coaster" is perhaps *the* metaphor for the ups and downs that make life worth living. The merry-go-round makes you merry and maybe a bit dizzy. But the roller coaster terrifies you, excites you, thrills you. You're the parent of an Aspie. You tell me: which of these two rides is more analogous to your day-to-day existence?

Knowing you're on an emotional roller coaster—each and every day—is what makes it so hard for me to shake you and say, "It's not about you. It's about your Aspie." Your Aspie is the one navigating the maze every day of her life. Sure, you're wandering through one too, trying to help. I understand that. But you're not the afflicted one. Your Aspie is. Don't lose sight of that.

So you cried at your niece's wedding because your Aspie may never experience marriage. Well, ignoring the statistic that more than half of all marriages in this country don't work out, who are you to feel sorry for someone just because they're not married? You're not the one struggling awkwardly with every relationship in your life. You're not the one who battles each day to learn all the difficult rules of socializing. Your Aspie's the one who does that.

So stop feeling sorry for yourself. It's not about you.

What's that? Your Aspie just verbally brutalized you when she stated an obvious fact that cut your inner emotional core to shreds? She made a blunt comment about something you're sensitive about? Your weight? Your crow's feet? Your job? Your divorce? Your close friend who's very sick? And when you responded like a wounded animal, your Aspie was surprised, looked at you, and said, "Well, I'm just telling you the truth."

Anger is not going to help you or your Aspie any more than self-pity will help you. Easy for me to say? Not really.

But the real question is, what are we trying to accomplish here? Answer: Whatever *you* can do to help the situation. You need to focus on *the actions you can take* to effect a positive change in your Aspie's behavior patterns to help her do better. When your Aspie does better, you feel better. And you do better. Life is better.

I'll give you all the accolades you want. Yes, you make daily sacrifices. Yes, you do so much for your Aspie. If you're a single mom, you deserve a special place in heaven. Maybe the father headed for the hills when he couldn't handle it, leaving you alone to teach your child, battle the schools, fight the medical establishment, deal with the bullying, go to work each day to support the family. You deserve so much admiration.

But Ms. Single Mom, you angel with the pit bull mentality, you know what? It's *still* not about you. I know you're tough. You deserve a big pat on the back, a parade down Main Street, and much more. But let's get back to work. Let's get back to doing positive things to help your Aspie maximize her success in a society not designed for someone with a brain that's "different." Together, let's give all people with the brains God gave them the best opportunity to maximize their independence, productivity, success, safety, and happiness. Everyone deserves that shot.

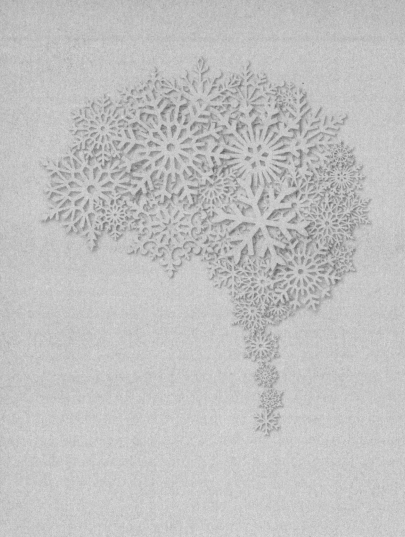

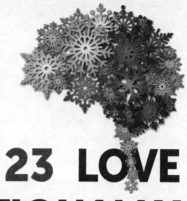

23 LOVE UNCONDITIONALLY

> Intense love does not measure,
> it just gives.
>
> — *Mother Teresa*

Helpful Hint: The greatest gift you can bestow upon your Aspie is the gift of unconditional love. That individual with the somewhat different brain absolutely needs your unconditional love.

Principle: If you think being loved is important to you, multiply that importance a thousand times over for Aspies, who feel tremendous anxiety at the thought that as a result of one of their actions, you might withhold your love. Because of their insecurity, what seems like a minor incident to you can cause them to doubt your love.

Imagine you're an Aspie. You're having a conversation with your mom. In the course of the conversation, she asked you if you had a good time yesterday with your dad. You tell her no. Your mom gives you a look. You're thinking: You asked me a question, I answered you honestly. Now you're shaking your head. I can see you're sad. I agree with what Jack Nicholson said in that movie we watched together: "You can't handle the truth!" If you didn't want the truth, why did you ask me in the first place?

Now you're looking at me funny. I'm not sure what you're thinking. That I don't love you? I love you. And you're the ones who are always hovering over me, following me everywhere, who won't let me escape to my room, who throw me into crowded rooms with lots of loud people, but I know that *you* love *me*. Or do you? Have I disappointed you too many times because my brain just can't keep up? Would you like to trade me for another child? With all of your rules and consequences, with your constantly telling me what to do and what not to do, with your always pointing out how I'm never doing things right, maybe you *don't* love me.

Action Plan: The most potent tool in your Aspertoolbox is *love*. When I think of my daughter, Rebecca, and how I love her so much and how blessed I am that she (and no one else) is my daughter—well, sometimes I wonder if she knows that. I know I say to her, "I love you all the time, no matter what." Love your Aspie all the way, all the time. And let him know you love him. Leave no doubt. (And let everyone else you love know it too.)

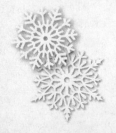

Thought from Rebecca

I love my dad unconditionally and would do anything to protect him. I am also blessed that I have him as my father. I love how he puts all his energy into a book with all intentions to learn more about my brain and how it works. I hope my dad will fully understand me one day the same way I completely understand him.

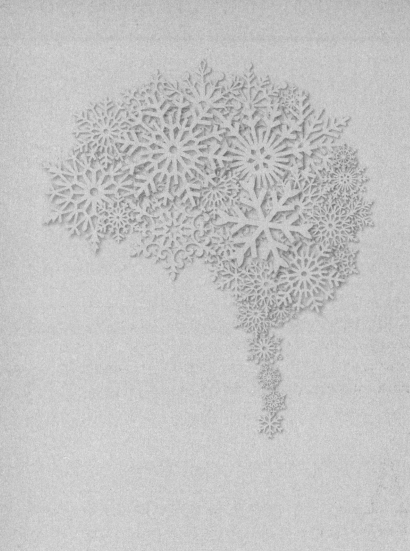

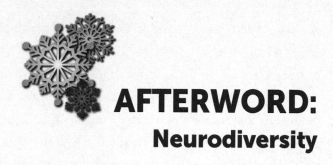

AFTERWORD:
Neurodiversity

Let us consider that we are all partially insane.
It will explain us to each other; it will unriddle
many riddles; it will make clear and simple many
things which are involved in haunting and
harassing difficulties and obscurities now.

—*Mark Twain*

A mericans accept diversity in many ways. We accept the
diversity of the color of one's skin. We accept the diversity of those with physical disabilities. We accept the
diversity of those immigrants who have legally joined the rest of
us immigrants here in the United States of America. We accept
the diversity of age, of religion, even of body type. In fact, it's the
law of the land. Discrimination on the basis of such differences
is illegal.

We are becoming more accepting of sexual diversity. The 2014
NFL draft will long be remembered for the selection of the first
openly gay college football player. When Michael Sam, a defensive

end from the University of Missouri, was finally picked in the seventh round, he wept with joy. Then the African-American Sam provided the NFL with another draft-day first when he gave his significant other, an emotional white male, a passionate kiss on the mouth. In that nationally televised moment, acceptance of diversity of sexual preference had finally come to the NFL.

God makes some of us dark, some of us light, and some of us in-between. He makes some of us tall and others "height challenged." So why is it so hard for us to accept the fact that God makes our brains different? Is it because there may not be a visual giveaway, like different-colored skin or, in the case of those who are disabled, a wheelchair or prosthesis? When it comes to different brains, it's time for everyone to stand up and say that we will no longer tolerate society's one-size-fits-all approach vis-a-vis education and the workplace. Asperger's syndrome is just one example of the vast array of different brains. There's the autistic brain, the ADHD brain, the OCD brain, the rest of the learning disorders brains, the psychological disorder brains (anxiety), and the psychiatric disorder brains (bipolar disorder, depression). God saw fit to give us all these different brains. Not better brains, not worse brains. Just different.

In many areas of the United States, if you add up the "minorities"—the Hispanics, Asian Americans, African Americans, you name the ethnicity—they demographically outnumber the Caucasian population. In other words, the once white majority is now the minority.

Just as ethnic diversity has become the rule, the same thing will happen with neurodiversity. The number of people with different brains is growing. If this trend continues, the neurotypicals, the so-called normal brains, will soon be in the neuro-minority (if they're not already).

And I believe the trend *will* continue. In fact, *it has to* if our collective brains are going to keep up with all the advances in technology and all the changes in how we perceive data and images. If you're a teenager today and your brain doesn't develop at least some form of ADHD, you might not be able to text on your smartphone while watching a video, listening to music, hearing (or pretending not to hear) your mom's instructions, checking out what's on TV, looking out the window, petting your dog, and so on. Your brain had better metamorphose to be able to take in all these stimuli and make some sense of them. In the same way that some Asperger's syndrome brains have an advantage over the neurotypical brain when it comes to, for example, focusing on numbers for long periods of time, certain types of brains are innately able to multitask. These brains have an advantage over the "old-fashioned" neurotypical brain, which could focus only on one thing at a time.

Back when we were teenagers, Paul Kaliades, Charlie Singer, and the rest of my pals spent countless hours playing stickball in the schoolyards of Jersey City. It was a relaxing way to spend an afternoon. Hardly any brain-related activity was involved, outside of the small talk of sports, girls, and arguing balls and strikes.[24]

Do you see teenagers playing stickball or any such relaxing activity today? I don't. Baseball has its loyal fans, but are today's ADHD teenagers willing or able to put up with its slow pace? Next time (or if) you go to a baseball game, locate a parent sitting with a teenage son or daughter, and see if the kid is watching the game or checking his phone. (The parent may be too.) In fact, when was the last time you were with someone who went fifteen minutes without texting, e-mailing, or checking some data or an app on his smartphone? Our digital communications are endless and relentless. Nobody's brain gets a rest these days.

Brains are changing in order to parallel the exponential changes in the Internet. It's not necessarily cause and effect. But look at the pace of change of civilization and technology. The printing press that Johannes Gutenberg developed during the Renaissance, sometime around 1450, changed the world radically, because it led to the first assembly-line mass production of books, but it didn't happen overnight. It took maybe fifty years. Another invention that changed society was television, and it took perhaps twenty years for the world to change its entertainment habits and become a living room TV society.

But it took the Internet less than a decade to overhaul everything: book publishing, newspapers, music, communication, education, television, sports, the way we read books and watch sports. There's no aspect of modern life that hasn't been disrupted by the Internet. And the disruption continues, with social media: Facebook, Twitter, Instagram, and Snapchat, to name just a few. Today the big changes take place over months, not centuries or decades.

The time has come not just to accept neurodiversity but to embrace it. What I originally thought would be a book about Asperger's syndrome turned out to be about everything I've learned about Aspies that applies to all types of brains, to all types of individuals to our entire society. I've learned that every brain is different. But as long as we share a common vision and certain basic values such as "Thou shalt not kill," "Do unto others," and so on, then "Every brain that is different" will be an accepted fact of life. Society will adapt to the differences in our brains just as it has to our other more easily recognizable differences. The educational system, workplace, and society will no longer be one size fits all. Each individual will have the opportunity to maximize his or her potential. And we will all be the better for it.

---

24 For those not familiar with Jersey City–style stickball, the strike zone is represented by a box drawn in chalk on a wall. On a close pitch, it's up to the batter and pitcher to decide if it was a strike or not (unless there's chalk on the ball to prove it).

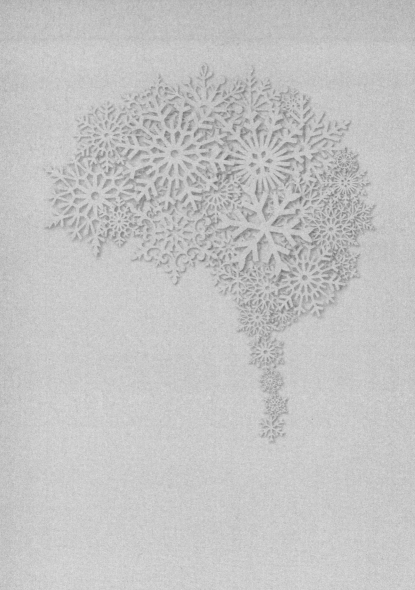

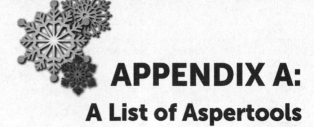

APPENDIX A:

A List of Aspertools

TOOL	USED BY	PURPOSE
Observation	Caregiver	Knowledge of Aspie's state of mind; useful for watching for signs of anxiety or triggers to ward off a meltdown.
Preparation	Caregiver	Prepares Aspies for any surprises or changes to their routines. Useful for getting ready for vacations, etc.
Patience	Caregiver	Gives Aspie time to process transitions, i.e., in conversations.
Training, role-playing	Caregiver and Aspie	Practicing social situations to avoid blow-ups and to teach Aspies not to be rude.
Using social stories/scripts	Caregiver	To foster success in social situations.
Consistency	Caregiver	Recommended in any area, because Aspies love consistency.
Admitting when you're wrong	Caregiver	Appeals to Aspie's sense of fairness.
Positive reinforcement; encouragement, smiles, hugs	Caregiver	Praise is one of the highest rewards for an Aspie.
Checklist	Aspie	Reminds them of daily tasks and prioritizes them; useful in time management.
System of rules, rewards, and consequences	Caregiver and Aspie	Encourages good behavior and discourages bad behavior.
Chart/pictorial/map	Caregiver and Aspie	Helps Aspies who are visual learners.
Posing questions in the proper manner	Caregiver	Easier to get them to agree to leaving comfort zone if given multiple choices.

Chunking	Caregiver and Aspie	Large/complicated projects intimidate Aspies. Breaking them down into smaller chunks enables the Aspie to handle the task.
Being specific with dates, hours, times	Caregiver	Ensures Aspies will comply with an assignment or request.
Harnessing hyper-interests	Caregiver	Aspies tend to focus very strongly on a few areas. These interests should be harnessed and encouraged if they are positive.
Explaining the meaning of idioms and colloquialisms	Caregiver	Many Aspies take idioms literally and must be taught what they mean.
Monitoring routines	Caregiver	Aspies do well when in a good routine; the trick is to help them set up the routine and see that they stay in it.
Teaching common sense and street smarts, Internet safety	Caregiver	Necessary for independence and survival. Establish rules.
Calmness, gentleness	Caregiver	Provides a quiet environment for Aspies to offset their hypersensitivity.
Creating relaxation techniques	Caregiver	Gives them the ability to calm themselves rather than relying on a professional.
Creating structure and positive activities	Caregiver	Aspies do well when their schedules are structured and when they engage in positive activities.
Forming Aspie circle	Caregiver and Aspie	Group of individuals who work together to check on Aspie's progress.
Compiling summary of medical history	Caregiver	Useful if Aspie visits a new specialist, as well as when applying for services.
Unconditional love	Caregiver	Perhaps the most important tool of all.

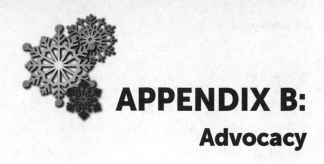

APPENDIX B:
Advocacy

Three simple rules in life:
If you don't go after what you want,
  you'll never have it.
If you don't ask, the answer will always be no.
If you don't step forward, you will always
  be in the same place.

—*Nora Roberts*

Principle: Even with the Internet, learning the ins and outs regarding learning disabilities is an uphill battle. Learning about disabilities and different brains is anything but static; it's up to you to keep up with this ever-changing landscape. If you've been doing that, then you know that the American Psychiatric Association did away with the diagnosis of Asperger's syndrome in its fifth edition of the *Diagnostic and Statistical Manual of Mental Disorders (DSM-5)*, which appeared in May 2013. People with Asperger's symptoms and behaviors are now evaluated under the broader diagnostic category of Autism Spectrum Disorder.

Why is this reclassification important? The *DSM* may indeed be, as the director of the National Institute of Mental Health (NIMH) and my Boston University School of Medicine classmate Tom Insel, MD, says, less of a bible for the field of mental disorders and more of a dictionary. Still, its diagnostic codes affect treatment decisions, insurance benefits, and government-mandated rights and supports, including what accommodations schools and employers must provide. If someone diagnosed with Asperger's doesn't qualify for an Autism Spectrum Diagnosis under the *DSM-5*, their families will have to fight harder to make sure they keep those services. Those necessary services and accommodations might even be denied altogether.

When I last spoke to Tom (who I admit at times is a lightning rod of controversy), we both agreed that it's probably not correct to merely list the terminology *Asperger's* as a type of autism. While Aspies are somewhere on the autism spectrum, they have characteristics that make them a bit different, maybe even unique.

The Aspie community is in an uproar about this loss of identity. People who have embraced the Asperger's label, who proudly call themselves Aspies, are wondering, "If this is taken away from us, who are we?" The change in nomenclature may most affect those Aspies who are not obviously struggling. For instance, some Aspies who are doing well in college, can pass socially, and can think their way through social situations may be off the radar of a lot of diagnosticians. But beneath it all they're still suffering, still in need of services on campus, still in need of accommodations. Those are people to be concerned about.

What should you, the parent of a child diagnosed with Asperger's, do about this big change? Here are some suggestions from the website of Dan Coulter, the author of *Life in the Asperger*

Lane. Adults diagnosed with Asperger's can take the same steps on their own behalf.

1. Review your child's current diagnosis information and any support they receive. Ask professionals and representatives of schools or other organizations that provide services about how long they plan to use an existing Asperger's diagnosis and how and when they will reevaluate individuals (or ask that you have them reevaluated) based on the new diagnosis criteria.

2. Stay informed. Many national and local Asperger's/ autism organizations are keeping a close watch on this issue and will be valuable sources of information. Each group will have its own perspective on the *DSM-5*, ranging from concerned to neutral to optimistic. [See Appendix C for more information on these resources.]

3. Be prepared to advocate to make sure the new autism diagnosis is interpreted and applied appropriately. If you're told your child doesn't qualify for a diagnosis under the *DSM-5* criteria, be ready to join with others to push to have that changed. While revising the specific wording of the new diagnosis may not be possible, you may be able to influence how the diagnosis is interpreted and applied by governmental, medical, or educational organizations. An organized effort by the Asperger's/ autism community could have enormous impact.

4. Be prepared to advocate for services. Even if your child is included in a diagnosis, you may have to work to ensure that the diagnosis entitles your child to the support he or she needs. Again, it will help to band together with

parents in similar situations or work through established groups.

5. If you have to fight, fight nice. Because you're not really fighting; you're advocating to help others understand your position, to see what you see. If you can establish common ground with the person across the table, with whom you are working together to ensure that those on the autism spectrum get the support and services they need, you're more likely to find solutions that work for everyone.

One important question is whether early intervention for children with Asperger's, which includes parent training, will be easier or harder to obtain under the new criteria.

Some people with Asperger's may fit under "social communication disorder" in the *DSM-5*. The manual is also adding "sensory sensitivity" to the autism spectrum criterion. This involves the extreme sensitivity to a person's environment discussed in the chapter on hypersenses.

Facts and Figures About Autism

When you look at the statistics about autism spectrum disorders, it's obvious that we need to direct resources to help deal with the issue. Let's start with this eye-popping statistic: According to a March 2014 study by the Centers for Disease Control and Prevention (CDC), autism alone is the "fastest growing developmental disability, with a 1,148 percent growth rate."

- One percent of the U.S. population of children between the ages of three and seventeen have an autism spectrum disorder.

- Prevalence is estimated at one in sixty-eight births.
- One million to 1.5 million Americans live with an autism spectrum disorder.
- Autism is the fastest-growing developmental disability: 1,148 percent growth rate.
- Ten to 17 percent annual growth.
- $60 billion annual cost.
- Sixty percent of costs are in adult services.
- Cost of lifelong care can be reduced by two-thirds with early diagnosis and intervention.
- In ten years, the annual cost will be between $200 billion and $400 billion.
- One percent of the U.K.'s adult population has an autism spectrum disorder.
- The cost of autism over the lifespan is $3.2 million per person.
- Only 56 percent of students with autism finish high school.
- The average per-pupil expenditure for educating a child with autism was estimated by SEEP to be over $18,000 in the 1999–2000 school year. This was nearly three times the expenditure for a typical regular-education student who did not receive special education services.
- The unemployment rate for people with disabilities was at 14 percent, compared with 9 percent for people without a disability. Additionally, during the same period, only 21 percent of all adults with disabilities participated in the labor force, compared with 69 percent of the population without disabilities.

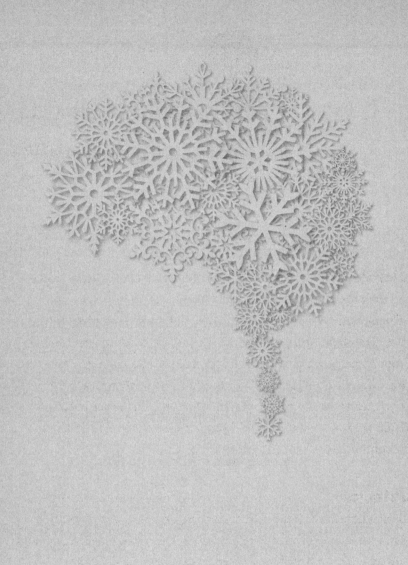

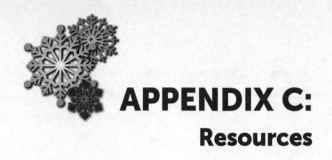

APPENDIX C:
Resources

Helpful Hint: Your Aspie probably won't ask for help—you'll be the one who needs to do that. So another one of your tasks is figuring out what help your Aspie needs and where to get that help. Research and locate the resources available to you and your Aspie at the local level as well as the national level. Get on the Internet and Google away! Search! Ask! Inquire! Because if you don't search or ask, you have no chance of receiving. Then fight the good fight to make sure Aspies get the help and accommodations that are rightfully theirs.

Principle: Despite all the publicity being heaped on learning disabilities, the resources available for families of Asperger's syndrome, autism spectrum, and other "different brain" individuals are woefully limited. Many parents of Aspies, especially the moms, have done noble battle with the system to obtain the accommodations and assistance their Aspies deserve and are legally entitled to. But even when the authorities want to help, the obstacle is the pervasive ignorance of the resources available for your Aspie (or for any other person with disabilities). You will fight a lot of battles—constant battles—and to win those battles you will need to arm yourself with knowledge. After all, the medical establishment, the educational establishment, the workplace establishment, and the government establishment have something in common. They're all tough.

Many more groups with a stake in this issue are good sources of information and support. The ones listed here are a good place to start. Some of these groups include The Autism Society of America and their state chapters, The Asperger Autism Spectrum Education Network (ASPEN), OASIS@MAAP, Autism Speaks, The Asperger/Autism Network (AANE), and Asperger Syndrome and High Functioning Autism Association (AHA).

This book isn't meant to be the ultimate referral source for Asperger's or high-functioning autism. If you do a Google search for "resources for Asperger's syndrome," the list of organizations goes on at length. If the bookstores and libraries in your area have limited resources on the subject, you'll have to go hunting online. Becoming part of a group that communicates well can provide many advantages if the individuals are positive-minded. Negativity does little good in general, and fighting the good fight for your Aspie is no exception. Do your homework and talk to others.

Here are a few more examples. The Center for Autism and Related Disorders (CARD) is at more than a few universities here in the tri-county area of Broward County, including Nova Southeastern University in Broward, Florida Atlantic University in Boca, and University of Miami. Available are e-mail groups and lists, Asperger's meet-up groups, Asperger's summer camps, as well as employment services and numerous qualified professionals such as psychologists, psychiatrists, ESE teachers, and educational programs. But let's face it: the system as it exists today is not as geared up as it should be to meet the needs of Aspies at any age level. But as Aspies enter adulthood, it gets especially lonely out there for their advocates.

Action Plan: Research, meet, talk, join, attend, speak, observe, read, watch, educate yourself and others, read some more, communicate, visit www.aspertools.com, and do Google searches. You're only as good as your information. And don't forget, you are not alone. Social media can be very helpful, and lots of groups exist.

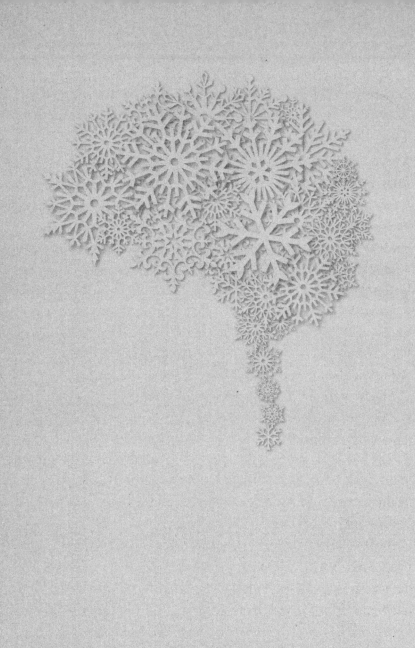